BURK JU
DEPART
SUNY H
750 E. AL
SYRACUSE, N.Y. 13210

D0566980

Post-Polio Syndrome

Post-Polio Syndrome

Edited by
Theodore L. Munsat, M.D.

Professor of Neurology
New England Medical Center
Tufts University Medical School
Boston, Massachusetts

With 15 Contributing Authors

Butterworth–Heinemann
Boston   London   Singapore   Sydney   Toronto   Wellington

Copyright © 1991 by Butterworth–Heinemann, a division of Reed Publishing (USA) Inc. All rights reserved.

No part of this publication may be reproduced, stored in a retrieval system, or transmitted, in any form or by any means, electronic, mechanical, photocopying, recording, or otherwise, without the prior written permission of the publisher.

Every effort has been made to ensure that the drug dosage schedules within this text are accurate and conform to standards accepted at time of publication. However, as treatment recommendations vary in the light of continuing research and clinical experience, the reader is advised to verify drug dosage schedules herein with information found on product information sheets. This is especially true in cases of new or infrequently used drugs.

 Recognizing the importance of preserving what has been written, it is the policy of Butterworth–Heinemann to have the books it publishes printed on acid-free paper, and we exert our best efforts to that end.

Library of Congress Cataloging-in-Publication Data
Post-polio syndrome / edited by Theodore L. Munsat ; with 15 contributing authors.
   p.   cm.
   Includes bibliographical references.
   ISBN 0-409-90153-9
   1. Poliomyelitis—Complications and sequelae.   I. Munsat, Theodore
L., 1930– .
   [DNLM: 1. Poliomyelitis—complications.   WC 555 P857]
   RC180.1.P67   1990
   616.8′35—dc20

                     90-1648

British Library Cataloguing in Publication Data
Post-polio syndrome.
   1. Man. Nervous system. Diseases I. Munsat, Theodore L.
   616.8
   ISBN 0-409-90153-9

Butterworth–Heinemann
80 Montvale Avenue
Stoneham, MA 02180

10 9 8 7 6 5 4 3 2 1

Printed in the United States of America

Contents

Contributing Authors

Patricia L. Andres, M.S., P.T.
Lecturer in Neurology
Tufts University School of Medicine
Research Physical Therapist
New England Medical Center
Boston, Massachusetts

Jack P. Antel, M.D.
Chair
Department of Neurology and
    Neurosurgery
McGill University
Montreal Neurological Institute
Montreal, Quebec, Canada

**Robert H. Brown, Jr., M.D.,
    D.Phil.**
Cecil B. Day Laboratory for
    Neuromuscular Disease
Neuroscience Center
Massachusetts General Hospital
Charlestown, Massachusetts

C. Brussock, M.S., P.T.
Neuromuscular Research Unit
Tufts New England Medical Center
Boston, Massachusetts

Neil R. Cashman, M.D.
Department of Neurology and
    Neurosurgery
McGill University
Montreal Neurological Institute
Montreal, Quebec, Canada

Marinos Dalakas, M.D.
Chief
Neuromuscular Diseases Section
National Institute of Neurological
    and Communicative Disorders
    and Stroke
National Institutes of Health
Bethesda, Maryland
Clinical Professor of Neurology
Georgetown University School of
    Medicine
Washington, D.C.

Richard Finkelman, M.D.
Neuromuscular Research Unit
Tufts New England Medical Center
Boston, Massachusetts

Lauro S. Halstead, M.D., M.P.H.
Director, Post-Polio Program
National Rehabilitation Hospital
Clinical Professor of Medicine
Georgetown University School of
    Medicine
Washington, D.C.

John J. Kelly, Jr., M.D.
Professor of Neurology
Tufts University School of Medicine
Senior Neurologist and Director of
    the EMG Laboratory
Tufts New England Medical Center
Boston, Massachusetts

Gini Laurie
Chair
International Polio Network
St. Louis, Missouri

Ricardo A. Maselli, M.D.
Department of Neurology
University of Chicago
Chicago, Illinois

Donald W. Mulder, M.D.
Emeritus Consultant
Department of Neurology
Mayo Clinic and Mayo Foundation
Emeritus Professor of Neurology
Mayo Medical School
Rochester, Minnesota

Dorothy Woods Smith, M.A., M.S., R.N.
Assistant Professor
University of Southern Maine
  School of Nursing
Portland, Maine
Doctoral Candidate
New York University
New York, New York

B. Thornell, P.T.A.
Neuromuscular Research Unit
Tufts New England Medical Center
Boston, Massachusetts

Robert L. Wollmann, M.D.
Department of Pathology
University of Chicago
Chicago, Illinois

Preface

Decades after their initial acute episode of poliomyelitis has passed, many survivors experience progressive weakness, fatigue, and pain. These symptoms have become so familiar and common that workers in the field have termed the disorder *post-polio syndrome*. Clarification of this syndrome might be a relatively simple task because the etiology, target organ, and sequelae of polio are well known. However, the syndrome continues to defy a full understanding.

Increasingly, post-polio syndrome has been shown to be an organic disorder of the motor unit. Although the actual mechanism of damage is still unclear, new research suggests that continuing reinnervation occurs after the acute attack of poliomyelitis subsides and that these new enlarged terminal motor units are less stable than the units they replace. As polio survivors recover and regain their normal physical activity levels, more and more functional activity is demanded of these restructured units and they become overburdened. Other motor units must now take over these activities and subsequently are also damaged. Thus, a cascading effect takes place and over several decades leads to the familiar symptoms of post-polio syndrome.

As many as 300,000 polio survivors are potential candidates for or are already experiencing the characteristic symptoms of post-polio syndrome. As the incidence and complexity of this disorder grows, the health-care profession will face considerable challenges in treatment and management. This book was undertaken to provide a review of our current understanding of the cause, symptoms, and treatment of post-polio syndrome from the perspective of basic scientists, clinicians, and therapists. Because there is presently no cure, treatment is based on an integrative approach that uses exercise and physical therapy to improve and strengthen motor function. In this book, clinical researchers examine the evidence they have gathered to support an etiology of post-polio syndrome based on electrophysiological changes, as well as on alterations in strength and muscle biopsy morphology. Andres outlines basic rehabilitation principles and the role of the physical therapist in managing the patient with post-polio syndrome. Finally, two polio survivors discuss the community resources available and the network support group for patients with post-polio syndrome.

While we are still a long way from having a definitive etiology for post-polio syndrome, this text provides our current knowledge and treatment for the disorder. It is my hope that physicians and therapists will find it a useful and enlightening resource when treating patients with post-polio problems.

T.L.M.

Chapter 1

Post-Polio Syndrome—Past, Present, and Future

Donald W. Mulder

The late sequelae of poliomyelitis were recognized in the past. A sketch from eighteenth dynasty Egypt records a man with a shortened, atrophied leg, often cited as an example of the late effects of polio, and a fifteenth century engraving by Bosch illustrates many of the characteristic deformities of patients with the residual weakness of polio [1]. The progression of weakness and atrophy in patients long after the acute episode of polio was reported more than 100 years ago, and patients with this characteristic weakness and atrophy were described in the early part of this century [2,3]. The introduction in 1955 of new and effective vaccines against polio brought about a dramatic reduction in the future incidence of the disease, such that polio with its attendant late progression of weakness was virtually forgotten until the recent recognition of increasing numbers of these patients. They now are being referred for their progressive weakness [4]. This rediscovery of a previously well-known syndrome has occasioned great anxiety in the half million survivors of the polio epidemics who now fear that their hard-won recovery is about to be lost, returning them, once again paralyzed, to the hospital.

Physicians trained during the past few decades know little of the polio epidemics and the emotional and physical impact they had on the patients and their families. This makes it difficult for them to appreciate the concerns of these patients and has led patients to feel abandoned by physicians. To render compassionate and effective care, physicians must understand the extraordinary ordeal polio patients experienced. This chapter describes how the polio epidemics were a unique experience for society, the paralyzed patient, and the treating physician.

THE POLIO EXPERIENCE AND SOCIETY'S ATTITUDES

Polio patients suffered the anxieties of an acute illness accentuated by the hysteria that accompanied the great polio epidemics. Their fears were heightened by the abrupt onset (often over one or two days) of paralysis, which made patients dependent on others, and the possibility that the illness would lead to respiratory failure or death. The stringent isolation of hospitalized patients, which deprived them of contact with family and friends, was often remembered as the most stressful aspect of the illness. This isolation was interpreted by many as abandonment. In fact, the fear of polio did lead to avoidance of patients, even by medical personnel.

Contemporary newspapers document the anxiety and mass hysteria remembered by patients who survived polio. Polio was "the sword of Damocles" that hung over every child and young adult. In the late summer and early fall of that era, newspapers ran headlines recording each new outbreak of polio. One typical small town newspaper reported in September and October of 1948 that because of the polio epidemic "the whole town must be closed as far as children are concerned. They must be kept strictly in their own yards" [5]. The town was sprayed with DDT and it was suggested that each family carry out an intensive spraying program of its own. An eight-year-old farmboy from the community developed polio during this epidemic. He remembers being brought to a large hospital where he was promptly isolated in a polio ward and was unable to see his parents or friends for two weeks. Forty years later, he still remembered the routine treatment with hot packs that were applied at "almost scalding temperature" [6].

This polio hysteria was nationwide and often included medical personnel. In a polio epidemic in Los Angeles during the summer of 1934, the stricken included 198 employees (16% of the student nurses) at the Los Angeles County Hospital [7]. These 198 patients were remarkable in that little fever or weakness occurred, and in only two of fifty-nine were abnormalities reported in the spinal fluid. Paul, in commenting on this epidemic, noted that hysterical cases encountered during polio epidemics could be identified "as having very little fever, a dearth of spinal fluid changes, little permanent weakness, and no deaths"—all characteristic of this epidemic among hospital employees. He noted that interpretation of this outbreak is difficult, but he agrees with the views of others that this and similar epidemics were caused by mass hysteria [1].

PATIENTS' ADAPTATION TO THE DISORDER

Once paralytic polio developed, many patients learned to compensate for and to adapt to their disability. They developed strong convictions about their illness while in the hospital with other polio patients. These convictions were initially believed because they brought the patients hope. They have remained unchanged even after the initial illness has subsided; and they dominate the post-polio patient's interpretation of his or her progressive weakness. Patients described their beliefs during the great epidemics in their medical histories, autobiographies, and biographies [8–24]. Physicians must be aware of these attitudes if they are to understand and care for the patient with post-polio weakness.

Compensatory Beliefs

Initially, patients struggled to compensate psychologically for their disability. One patient wrote,

> We have a slowly forming new attitude to life in the world. Again, we have to learn to compensate gradually for what we do not have by what we have. . . . I had somehow to encompass with my mind the limitation of my body [22].

This attempt to attain maximal function both physically and psychologically took many years and great physical and emotional effort. The patient's adaptation was often accompanied by the belief that anything was possible if you only tried hard enough. This in turn led to the patient's almost superhuman struggles to achieve in many spheres; many patients who had paralytic polio later became successful in many endeavors [11,13,17].

A related belief held by patients who successfully compensated was that they could only recover. One patient wrote, "Once the initial attack is over, there is no question of the sufferer's becoming worse. Always we improve and the chances are good that we shall regain 100% mobility" [20]. Another wrote, "The only direction a patient can move is toward improvement and perhaps complete recovery" [16]. This belief in inevitable recovery was often accompanied by a belief that it was the positive spirit of the individual patient that was responsible for the recovery. A patient wrote, "Just keep trying to strengthen your muscles and you too will walk" [20]. Another wrote, "This improvement is a thrilling thing, and although it may be a natural process, you can't help feeling but that your personal contributions are not small" [12]. Often associated with this belief in recovery was a denial by patients, family members, and physicians of the extent of the patient's residual disability.

Distrust of the Medical Establishment

Distrust of physicians began early in many who had paralytic polio. It often began when the patient noticed confusion on the part of his or her physicians— a confusion that often interfered with the treatment of the patient. Many patients were initially misdiagnosed or mismanaged. One patient wrote, "Thus, I ran for the first time into that difference of opinion between doctors of which I was to see a great deal. Granted that medicine is an art as much as a science, by what signs is a patient to know which doctor is a better artist?" [16]. Another patient wrote, "The extent of bracing depended on which orthopedist was on duty that month" [15]. Treatment or lack of treatment often depended on the patient's locale or physician. Distrust of the medical establishment was only abetted by the prolonged hospitalization that usually accompanied the illness. During such hospitalizations many patients became aware of the errors and foibles of the best of our medical institutions. Patients' distrust of physicians has continued and makes the physician's role in the care of patients with post-polio sequelae particularly difficult.

TREATMENT DURING THE EPIDEMICS

A review of the customary diagnosis and treatment of poliomyelitis in the first half of this century reinforces one's sympathy with the patient's concern [25,26]. For much of this century, diagnosis was dependent on the clinical history and examination, with a spinal fluid examination for confirmation. It was only as the epidemics were winding down that specific viral studies became readily available [1]. Understandably, the diagnosis was often overlooked during non-epidemic periods. During epidemics polio was commonly overdiagnosed. At these times, paralysis of any kind was often diagnosed as polio, including peripheral neuropathy, stroke, brain or spinal cord tumors, multiple sclerosis, and hysterical paralysis. Once the diagnosis of polio had been established, it was difficult to change because of the generous financial support given to the victims of polio but not to those with other forms of paralysis.

Many specific therapies were advocated, including drugs such as strychnine, Prostigmin (neostigmine), urocholine, curare, cobra venom, and various anti-biotics [1,25,26]. Most of these preparations were given orally, but some were given by injection, even intrathecally. The reports of their efficacy were based on anecdotal information but were propounded with certitude. A commonly advocated therapy was radiography of the muscles or spinal cord [26,27].

In the twentieth century it became commonplace to splint and cast patients. Large depositories of splints were placed in locations throughout the country and were made available during polio epidemics. Paralyzed patients lay in posterior plaster body casts for months at a time. Prolonged casting led to disuse and atrophy of muscles not already affected by the disease [28]. Paul reported that during the epidemic among Los Angeles County Hospital employees in 1934, 74% of the patients had one or more extremities splinted and 46% were immobilized on a Bradford frame. The interns on the ward reported that after encasing one or more limbs in a cast, the patient's symptoms often worsened [1].

Orthopedic surgery was used extensively for fixing joints, lengthening and shortening extremities, increasing circulation to affected limbs, and transferring muscles in affected limbs [26,28]. School-age patients spent every summer in orthopedic hospitals to undergo such procedures.

In 1951, Irish physician C.J. McSweeney described the treatment of poliomyelitis by the medical establishment of the United States after visiting polio centers throughout the country [28]. He noted that therapy varied from state to state. This was particularly true of surgical therapy, which was used in some centers during the acute stage of the illness, or shortly thereafter. Specifically, tracheostomy was being used in more than half of the patients with bulbar palsy on the West Coast but in only 6% of the patients with bulbar palsy elsewhere.

Sister Kenny, an Australian nurse, had developed her own therapy. This therapy was the center of controversy in most centers. The almost universal distrust of the medical establishment by patients with polio did not extend to Sister Kenny. The treatment she proposed for acute polio was the application of warm moist heat (wool packs) to the affected areas in combination with early activity. This was contrary to the opinion of many medical professionals who advocated casting or splinting. Sister Kenny undertook a worldwide crusade advocating her system of treatment. Much of the crusade was carried out in the newspapers. Victor Cohn provides an interesting description of it in *Sister Kenny: The Woman Who Challenged the Doctors* [29].

The controversy about Sister Kenny's treatment program attracted attention to polio and to the confusion about its treatment, both in Australia and worldwide. Sister Kenny's achievements led to the improved care of polio patients. Her achievements included the substitution of optimistic activity for immobilization, and the recognition that when a limb is placed in a splint for a prolonged period it loses its function, a physiologic state she called *alienation*.

Franklin D. Roosevelt

The biographies of eminent people who had polio illustrate the compensatory attitudes and adaptations of patients with the illness [11,13,17]. Franklin D. Roosevelt's polio with severe residual paralysis is well documented [11]. At age 39 he became paralyzed over a twenty-four-hour period while vacationing at his summer home on an island off the coast of New Brunswick. The illness was originally diagnosed as a blood clot on the spinal cord. Physical examination at that time revealed paralysis of his legs and weakness of both arms. Two weeks later, the diagnosis was changed to indicate polio, and he was brought, still paralyzed, to New York City for hospitalization. During the next few months, contractures of his knees and right foot developed and were treated with plaster casts.

Roosevelt spent the next eight years (1921 to 1928) adapting to his physical limitations. He sought treatment first in and around New York City and later in Warm Springs, Georgia. In 1926 Roosevelt bought the hotel and resort in Warm Springs and converted it to a polio treatment center. He spent much of his time there attempting to regain his ability to walk unaided, and although he achieved only minor improvement, it was still of great significance to him. By 1928 he had learned to simulate walking by using braces and a cane while holding on to an aide's arm. When Roosevelt re-entered the political arena that year he usually appeared in public either seated or standing, and only rarely walking with support. He was never photographed in a wheelchair or being carried, although these were his common methods of transportation.

Gallagher described how Roosevelt adapted to his illness in *FDR's Splendid Deception* [11]. Gallagher had also had paralytic polio and had been a patient at Warm Springs. Thus, he has unusual insight into the response of patients with polio. The title of his book is provocative: who was being deceived? On first glance it appears to have been the public. However, if the public was deceived, it must have been willingly. Many people helped carry Roosevelt in the White House, on his weekly fishing trips, and on his political trips. Many more must have witnessed this [10]. Roosevelt traveled widely by train, and in his political campaigns he spoke from the rear of his observation car. Anyone who watched him struggle through the door of the car with his cane and braces, leaning on the arm of one of his sons, would realize he had a severe disability.

Gallagher suggests that FDR was deceiving himself. It is probable that he, like others with severe post-polio disability, thought of himself as able-bodied and did not wish to have pictures or comments in the press that indicated otherwise. Missy LeHand, his secretary and confidante, reported that Roosevelt always believed that if he had spent one more year at Warm Springs, he would have learned how to walk with only a single brace and no cane or arm assist. When reviewing an article for *Liberty* magazine that greatly upset him, he is reported to have said, "This magazine says I never recovered from infantile paralysis. Never recovered! I have only never recovered the full use of my knees. Correct that!" [9]. Of course it was true that he no longer had acute polio, but even the most casual observer could see that he still had severe muscle weakness that affected more than his knees.

Roosevelt's disabilities increased as he aged. In his last year he had difficulty lighting a cigarette, holding a cup of coffee, and driving a car. Thus, he clearly had progression of his weakness. As with other post-polio patients, there were many apparent causes for his increasing weakness, in addition to his residual polio. These included inactivity, cardiac failure, and hypertension. His family had accepted the image he portrayed and found it difficult to accept his increased disability. Gallagher reports that Roosevelt complained to his wife that he would be unable to live out a normal life span because of his weakness, saying, "I can't even walk across the room to get my circulation going." Mrs. Roosevelt interpreted his progressive symptoms as psychological, writing to a friend that FDR was giving way to invalidism [11].

APPROACH TO THE PATIENT WITH POST-POLIO SYNDROME

A review of the medical histories, biographies, and autobiographies of patients who developed severe disability from polio reveals that they adopted firm convictions about their disease and recovery. As physicians, we must be aware of these convictions if we are to treat their later disabilities successfully. Polio survivors often believe that they can only improve, and that this improvement is primarily related to their willingness to engage in exercise. To them, improvement is more related to the spirit than to medication. Associated with this conviction is a denial of the extent of the disability—a denial often shared by the family. Furthermore, the confusion of physicians during the great epidemics suggests to patients that we can be of little help today.

These convictions, which were invaluable when the patients were young and vigorous, become a liability when aging and progressive weakness supervene. Patients, who had adapted to muscle weakness through great physical and emotional effort, are unable to continue functions they had regained. They cannot accept that they do not continue to improve, and many become depressed. They may consult their physicians; however, most remember that earlier physicians had been misdirected or even wrong about polio and its treatment. They hesitate to bring their concerns to their physicians, and when they do, they frequently find that physicians do not share their convictions. Instead of being concerned about the progressive weakness, physicians are amazed at their ability to adapt to their obvious motor disability. This disability is often denied by patients, who report that they were perfectly recovered except for some minor defect, just as Roosevelt had insisted that his only difficulty was in his knees. The result of such confrontation is often a belief by patients that the physician does not understand or is not sympathetic to their disability, whereas physicians cannot understand why the patient is concerned about what seems to be only a slight worsening of an overwhelming disability.

It is imperative in our treatment of patients with late sequelae of polio that we take into account the illness they have overcome. Physicians who examine such patients are often reassured that they do not have a new neurologic disorder such as amyotrophic lateral sclerosis. They may imply to patients that their new weakness is of no significance and is only related to their previous polio. This is not reassuring to patients who are deathly afraid that the acute episode of polio they had many years ago may recur. The proper care of patients with post-polio syndrome requires that physicians understand the acute polio epidemics and patients' responses to this overwhelming illness. The physician should be aware that many patients who have had paralytic polio will later develop weakness and fatigue (post-polio syndrome). Some will develop progressive muscular atrophy and weakness. The subsequent chapters of this monograph discuss these syndromes and their therapy.

REFERENCES

1. Paul JR. A history of poliomyelitis. New Haven, Conn: Yale University Press, 1971.
2. Mulder DW, Rosenbaum RA, Layton DD Jr. Late progression of poliomyelitis or forme fruste amyotrophic lateral sclerosis? Mayo Clin Proc 1972;47:756–61.

3. Meyerding HW. Mayo Clinic archives report of the Orthopedic Department for 1925.
4. Codd MKB, Kurland LT. Polio's late effects. In: 1986 Medical and health annual. Chicago: Encyclopedia Britannica, 1985, pp 249–52.
5. Tri-county Record, Rushford, Minn, August 27, 1987.
6. Rustad D. Personal communication, 1988.
7. Gilliam AG. Epidemiological study of an epidemic, diagnosed as poliomyelitis, occurring among the personnel of the Los Angeles County General Hospital during the summer of 1934. Public Health Bull No. 240, 1938, pp 1–90.
8. Alexander L. The iron cradle. New York: Thomas Y Crowell, 1954.
9. Asbell B. F.D.R.'s extra burden. Am Heritage 1973;4:21–5.
10. Brown W. Aid to four presidents. Am Heritage 1955;2:66–96.
11. Gallagher HG. F.D.R.'s splendid deception. New York: Dodd Mead, 1985.
12. Goldman RL. Even the night. New York: Macmillan, 1947.
13. Haley KHD. The first Earl of Shaftesbury. Oxford: Clarendon Press, 1968.
14. Hawkins LC. The man in the iron lung. Garden City, N.Y.: Doubleday, 1956.
15. Lake L. Each day a bonus. Salt Lake City: Deseret Book Company, 1971.
16. LeComte L. The long road back. Boston: Beacon Press, 1957.
17. Lockhart JG. Memoirs of the life of Sir Walter Scott, Vol. 1. Edinburgh, Scotland: A and C Black, 1882.
18. Marshall A. I can jump puddles. Cleveland: The World Publishing Company, 1956.
19. Marugg J. Beyond endurance. London: Rupert Hart-Davis, 1955.
20. Opie J. Over my dead body. New York: EP Dutton, 1957.
21. Ostenso M. And they shall walk. New York: Dodd Mead, 1943.
22. Plagemann B. My place to stand. London: Victor Gollancz, 1950.
23. Walker T. Rise up and walk. New York: EP Dutton, 1950.
24. Garrison FH. Sir Walter Scott's lameness. JAMA 1919;73:709–10.
25. Wechsler IS. A textbook of clinical neurology with an introduction to the history of neurology, 5th ed. Philadelphia: WB Saunders, 1943, p 109.
26. Weinstein L. Diagnosis and treatment of poliomyelitis. Med Clin North Am 1948; Sept (Boston): 1377–1402.
27. Fishbein M, Salmonsen E, Hektoen L. A bibliography of infantile paralysis, 2nd ed. Philadelphia: Lippincott, 1951.
28. McSweeney CJ. A visit to poliomyelitis centres in the U.S.A. Ir J Med Sci 1951;6:65–73.
29. Cohn V. Sister Kenny: the woman who challenged the doctors. Minneapolis: University of Minnesota Press, 1975.

Chapter 2

Molecular Biology of Poliovirus—A Review

Robert H. Brown, Jr.

Poliovirus is a neurotropic RNA virus that causes paralytic poliomyelitis. As outlined in Garrison's *History of Neurology* [1], the scourge of paralytic poliomyelitis is evident in some of the oldest records of human history. Egyptian murals more than 3,000 years old depict probable residual effects of poliovirus in the priest Ruma, who is illustrated using a cane because of a shortened, atrophied right leg. The first clinical description of the illness was by Underwood in 1789. Duchenne and later Charcot and Joffroy presented the first histopathological descriptions of the lesions of poliomyelitis in the anterior horn of the spinal cord in the mid-nineteenth century. While the epidemic nature of poliomyelitis was first emphasized by Medin in 1890 [2], the communicable nature of the poliovirus was not described until 1907. Discovery of the virus as a filterable, transmissible agent was reported in 1908 by Landsteiner and Popper [3] and in 1909 by Flexner and Lewis [4,5]. Careful pathological studies by Bodian and colleagues in the late 1940s and early 1950s confirmed the high degree of motor specificity of lesions of poliovirus in the human neuraxis [6]. A central advance in understanding the poliovirus was its propagation in cell culture, for which Enders and Weller received the Nobel prize. With the development and widespread use of successful vaccinations by Sabin and Salk, poliovirus was largely eradicated from Western society. Nonetheless, investigations of this virus and the molecular basis for its pathological effects have continued for several reasons. This virus is representative of the large class of picornaviruses and is relatively easy to propagate and study. Its simplicity makes it an ideal model in which to analyze the processes governing viral gene replication and expression. Because of its devastating effects on host cells, it is an excellent tool for the analysis of both viral and cellular protein synthesis and the mechanisms whereby viruses impair cell function. Because its receptor has recently been cloned and partially characterized, poliovirus is likely to be used widely to analyze viral-receptor interactions. Finally, as reviewed elsewhere in this book, the epidemic of new neuromuscular dysfunction years after stable recovery from old poliomyelitis has revived clinical interest in the poliovirus, as has the recognition that an understanding of the motor specificity of the virus may provide insight into other motor-specific disorders, such as amyotrophic lateral sclerosis. This chapter is intended to provide a broad overview of the molecular nature of the poliovirus and mechanisms whereby it is injurious to selected mammalian cells.

BASIC STRUCTURE OF POLIOVIRUS

The Viral Coat

At about 30 nanometers in diameter, this RNA virus is relatively small (hence the name *pico*rnavirus [7]). The virus lacks a lipid coat or capsule but has a protein coat believed to have the shape of a polyhedron with twenty faces. This coat, or capsid, is composed of sixty copies of each of four viral proteins (VP), designated VP1, VP2, VP3 and VP4 (see Figures 2.1–2.3). The structure of the capsid in the mature virion has been elegantly analyzed by x-ray crystallography [8]. VPs1–3 each have a central core with regions that form both externally and internally directed projections from the capsid. VP4 is located

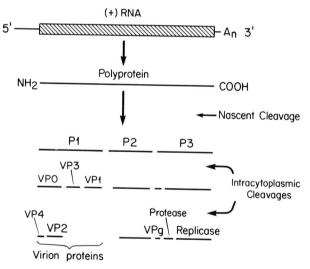

FIGURE 2.1   *Synthesis of poliovirus proteins. The poliovirus RNA is positive stranded and monocistronic. It is directly translated into a large polyprotein that subsequently is cleaved into smaller proteins as indicated. P1 is cleaved to form VP0, VP1, and VP3; VP0 subsequently is cleaved to form VP2 and VP4. VPg, polioviral replicase and viral proteases arise from P2 and P3. (Modified with permission from Watson et al. [36] and Luria et al. [7].)*

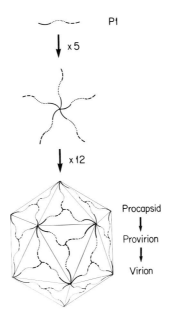

Procapsid
↓
Provirion
↓
Virion

FIGURE 2.2 *Morphogenesis of poliovirus. During polioviral capsid formation, five copies of P1 form a pentamer linked at the VP1 end (solid line). Twelve pentamers form the icosohedral procapsid, which has 20 faces. The immature provirion is formed when newly synthesized polioviral RNA packaged within the procapsid is converted to the mature virion by cleavage of VP0 (dashed line) into VP2 and the internally located VP4. (Modified with permission from Watson et al. [36].)*

exclusively within the capsid. Sequence analysis suggests that the three known serotypes or strains of poliovirus have very similar amino acid sequences within the cores of the proteins; sequence differences are most pronounced in regions that form the projections. These crystallographic studies also suggest that sites recognized by antibodies that neutralize poliovirus are all located on the viral surface and occur predominantly in a few restricted regions.

The Poliovirus Genome

The poliovirus genome is a single-stranded RNA of approximately 7,400 nucleotides that have been fully sequenced [9,10]. This is said to be a positive strand because after penetration into the host cell it can immediately be translated into protein without an intermediary complementary DNA or RNA. Poliovirus RNA is polyadenylated at its 3' end. At the 5' terminus it is covalently linked to a protein VPg via a phosphodiester bond at the terminal uridine (-U-U-VPg). VPg is a poliovirus peptide of twenty-two amino acids that may have a role in initiation of polioviral RNA synthesis. Within nine

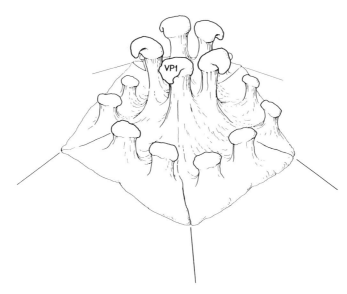

FIGURE 2.3 *Receptor-binding "canyon." This view of a vertex of the polioviral capsid demonstrates the depression or canyon that lies between the prominent epitopes of VP1 centrally and regions of VP1, VP2, and VP3 laterally. The receptor binding site is believed to reside within the floor of the canyon where it is inaccessible to large structures such as Fab fragments of antibody; however, it is accessible to smaller proteins such as one of the domains of the poliovirus receptor.*

nucleotides of the 5' end of the RNA, there is a twenty-seven–nucleotide stem and loop structure in the RNA of uncertain significance; the loop configuration suggests a recognition or regulatory function. In at least one strain of poliovirus (Lansing type 2) the 5' noncoding region contains seven AUGs followed by in-frame termination codons. The AUG that initiates translation of the viral proteins is downstream [11].

LIFE CYCLE OF THE POLIOVIRUS

Adsorption and Entry—The Poliovirus Receptor

The initial step in poliovirus infection is adsorption of virus to the surface of the host cell. Much data suggests that adsorption is both tissue and species specific, and is likely to be receptor mediated. Thus, homogenates of susceptible tissues such as primate brain or spinal cord are capable of adsorbing polioviral infectivity, whereas homogenates of insusceptible tissues are not. Brain homogenates from humans and monkeys adsorb infectivity, whereas those from insusceptible species such as mice do not [12]. (The principal exception is the Lansing strain of poliovirus type 2, which produces lytic infection and fatal paralysis in mice [13].) Binding activity appears to be enhanced in brain fractions enriched in synaptic proteins [14]. Poliovirus-resistant cells may support lytic polio infections if the polioviral RNA is delivered in coats of viruses that infect the cells [15]; in this circumstance, the host cells support a single cycle of poliovirus replication. Recently, poliovirus-resistant mouse L cells have been rendered polio sensitive by stable transfection with human cDNA, which encodes a surface molecule apparently able to bind poliovirus [16]. Analysis of poliovirus binding to mouse-human hybrid cells indicates that a poliovirus-binding protein is encoded by human chromosome 19 [17,18], probably in the region 19q12–q13.2 [19].

Biochemical analysis of the poliovirus receptor has historically been difficult. Whereas some parameters, such as pH and cation sensitivity of binding or density of binding sites (approximately 10^3 to 10^4 per cell), were readily determined, and whereas receptor activity has been solubilized [20], purification has been hindered because traditional methods destroy poliovirus binding activity [21]. These points notwithstanding, remarkable progress has been achieved in understanding this receptor largely through the use of monoclonal antibodies (MoAbs) and gene-cloning methods. Minor and colleagues described two MoAbs that block polioviral binding to Hep2c cells [22]. Nobis et al. generated MoAb D171, which protects HeLa cells from infection with all three serotypes of poliovirus, but not from other types of viruses [23]. More recently, Shepley, Sherry, and Weiner produced MoAb AF3, which inhibits infection of HeLa cells with poliovirus type 2 and detects a 100-kilodalton protein in Western blots of cell lines and tissues susceptible to poliovirus [24]. AF3 immunostained regions such as the reticular formation known to be heavily damaged by poliovirus infection in vivo; staining was prominent over neuronal cell bodies but not axons or white matter.

Recently, major progress in understanding the poliovirus receptor was achieved with its cloning and sequencing by Mendelsohn, Wimmer, and Racaniello [25]. These authors have cloned two forms of the poliovirus receptor encoding proteins of 43,000 and 45,000 daltons; the differences in size arise from variations in the cytoplasmic portions of the molecule. Sequence analysis (Figure 2.4) indicates the presence of a 24–amino acid transmembrane domain and three potential extracellular loops arising from cysteine pairs. Each of these three domains shows a high degree of homology to conserved regions of members of the immunoglobulin superfamily. The greatest homologies in domains 1, 2, and 3 were respectively to human immunoglobulin (Ig) lambda chains, human leukocyte antigen (HLA) class II histocompatibility antigens, and the mouse neural cell adhesion molecule (N-CAM). The latter observation is particularly striking in view of the simultaneous reports that the major group of rhinoviruses bind to another Ig superfamily member, the intercellular adhesion molecule, or I-CAM [26–28]. Analogously, human immunodeficiency virus (HIV) binds to the protein CD4, another Ig family member (Figure 2.4).

Expression of the polioviral receptor gene does not closely correlate with the tissue tropism of the virus. Northern analysis detected RNA for the polio-

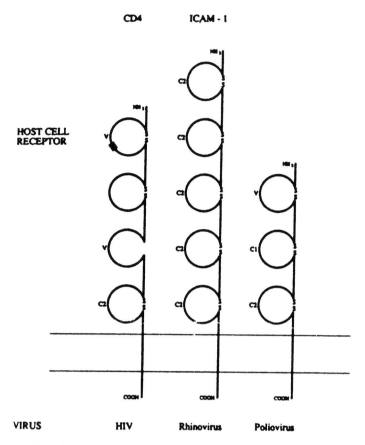

FIGURE 2.4   *Putative structures of receptors for human immunodeficiency virus (HIV), rhinovirus, and poliovirus. Homologous structures of the receptors for HIV (CD4), rhinovirus (I-CAM), and poliovirus are illustrated demonstrating domains that share homology with members of the immunoglobulin superfamily. (Reprinted with permission from White and Littman [27].)*

virus receptor in tissues such as human kidney, which do not support poliovirus replication. This result suggested that in insusceptible tissues the cellular mRNA does not give rise to receptor protein, possibly because the mRNA is not translated or because it fails to undergo an essential posttranslational modification.

Precisely how the poliovirus engages the poliovirus receptor remains unclear. It is striking that numerous immunologically distinct strains of the closely related rhinoviruses bind a common rhinovirus receptor [29]. This has suggested that the picornavirus receptor binding regions are likely to be similar in the different strains of rhinovirus and possibly protected or inaccessible to those antibodies that define the viral strains as dissimilar. Rossman and colleagues have emphasized that antibodies that neutralize picornaviruses bind the hypervariable regions of the capsid proteins, particularly on VP1, that protrude from the vertices of the virus capsid as shown in Figure 2.3 [30]. Surrounding these protruding vertices are indented regions with highly conserved amino acid sequences. Rossman et al. have hypothesized that these conserved regions forming the floor of the protected "canyon" around the pentamer vertices are candidate foci for the receptor binding sites. As reviewed by White and Littman [27], in rhinovirus the canyon dimensions (25 A deep by 12–30 A wide) preclude binding by antibody Fab (diameter 35 A) but not by the loop domains of the immunoglobulin family members, which are about 20 A in diameter.

The attachment of poliovirus to the cell surface is followed by entry of the viral RNA into the cell. This process apparently alters the structure of the capsid, as suggested by changes in antigenicity of the capsid after loss of the viral RNA. At least one component of this process must occur at the cell surface; modified polio virions without RNA can be recovered from the cell after adsorption. Data also suggest that poliovirus may gain entry to the cell by receptor-mediated endocytosis [31]. Adenosine triphosphate–dependent acidification of these vessicles is essential for RNA translocation into the host cell cytoplasm [32]. After RNA entry into the cell there is an "eclipse" phase prior to the emergence of new, infectious poliovirus.

Viral and Cellular Protein Synthesis

During the eclipse phase, several processes must occur for successful release of infectious virus: inhibition of function of the host cell, transcription of viral mRNA, replication of the viral genome, morphogenesis of the new virion, and release from the cell. For poliovirus this entire process requires only about five hours. Because the poliovirus RNA is positive stranded and can be directly transcribed, the eclipse period is shorter in poliovirus than in many other animal viruses, but is considerably slower than in bacteriophages. The effect of poliovirus on host cell protein synthesis is dramatic. Within two hours, host protein synthesis is reduced to less than 20% of baseline levels. The reduction in cellular protein synthesis is mediated by a protein synthesized by the poliovirus mRNA. This inhibitory protein does not alter the host cell mRNA. Rather, it acts to prevent binding of cellular mRNA to ribosomes by inactivating a host cell translation initiation factor, eIF-4B [33]. Eukaryotic cellular mRNA (and indeed that of many viruses) is modified after transcription to have a polyadenylated tail at the 3′ end and a "cap" at the 5′ end, which includes 7-methylguanosine linked to the RNA by three phosphates. It is to this cap that eIF-4B binds to initiate cellular mRNA translation. By cleaving eIF-4B, the poliovirus protein effectively terminates host cell protein synthesis. In contrast to the cellular mRNA, the mRNA of poliovirus is not capped; it has recently been reported that poliovirus mRNA may bind to ribosomes via one or more essential untranslated region in the 5′ end of the molecule [34–36]. Thus, the proteolytic disruption of eIF-4B by poliovirus produces selective inhibition of host cell but not polioviral protein synthesis.

As noted above, there are four poliovirus proteins in the capsid; in addition, the poliovirus genome codes for at least four additional proteins, including the 5' terminal protein VPg, two proteases, and an RNA-dependent, RNA polymerase known as replicase. The translational efficiency of the poliovirus mRNA is modified by several factors. There are cis-acting elements in the 5'-noncoding region that inhibit translation of the RNA; in contrast, transacting factors in host cells apparently enhance translation [11]. It is a striking property of poliovirus that the mRNA is monocistronic (Figure 2.1); the mRNA has only one coding region that encodes a single large precursor protein of about 240 kilodaltons from which the mature proteins are generated by cleavage first into three intermediate proteins P1, P2, and P3, and then into the mature viral proteins. Thus, as described below, one of the intermediate proteins, P1, encompasses the capsid proteins VP1–4. P2 and P3 give rise to replicase, VPg, and two viral proteases. The proteases cleave the precursor polyprotein at specific amino acid groups such as glutamine-glycine bonds. Because the poliovirus mRNA is positive stranded, synthesis of these proteins may begin immediately after entry of the mRNA into the host cell. The cleavage into P1, P2, and P3 is said to be nascent because it occurs almost immediately after the bonds to be cleaved are formed. Later cleavages of the resulting proteins are described as intracytoplasmic because they occur following release of the proteins from the ribosomes. At least one cleavage (VP0 to VP2 and VP4) does not occur until the final stage of maturation of the viral capsid.

Viral RNA Replication

The poliovirus RNA replicates via a negative strand of RNA ([−] RNA) or replicative intermediate formed from the positive strand ([+] RNA) through the action of the replicase. Essential to replicase function is the -U-U-VPg moiety, noted above, which serves as a primer by binding to the poly A region of the 3' end of the (+) RNA. Because the 5' end of the (+) RNA is covalently linked to VPg through a -U-U- residue, the 3' end of the newly formed (−) RNA replicative intermediate will end in -A-A. Thus, when new (+) RNA is made from this (−) RNA, -U-U-VPg can again serve as a primer; it will now reside at the 5' end of the resulting (+) RNA [37]. During a typical infection, there will be at least three species of RNA present: (+) RNA, (−) RNA, and a fraction that is a double helix of (+) and (−) RNA. Approximately four hours after infection with a single polio virion, an infected cell will have about 600 replicative intermediates, each producing five or so chains of polioviral RNA per minute or a total of 3,000 new molecules of polioviral RNA per minute. Thus, in about the fifth hour after the initial infection, some $1-2 \times 10^5$ new copies of viral RNA are produced.

Viral Morphogenesis and Cell Lysis

Morphogenesis of the mature poliovirion is complex. The capsid proteins are all derived from the precursor protein P1, which is cleaved initially into VP1, VP3, and VP0. When this cleavage occurs, a pentamer is formed from five clusters of the resulting VP1, VP3, and VP0 proteins. Twelve of these pentamers then aggregate to form a procapsid with twenty faces and twelve pentameric peaks (Figure 2.2). When poliovirus RNA enters the procapsid, the resulting provirus is converted to mature virus by cleavage of VP0 to VP2 and VP4. Presumably this last proteolytic step confers a final change in the virion structure that seals in and protects the viral RNA. P1, VP1, and ultimately VP4 are linked to tetradecanoic acid (myristic acid), which may stabilize interactions with host cell membranes during morphogenesis and infection [38].

The precise sequence of events leading to the final "burst" or lysis of the poliovirus-infected cell is not well defined. It seems likely that lysis is primarily a consequence of inhibition of cellular metabolism. Whether there are specific effects of the 2×10^5 virions on membrane permeability and integrity has not been reported.

NEUTRALIZATION AND VIRULENCE

It has been recognized for more than two decades that there are three major serotypes of poliovirus, as defined by neutralization by different antisera. Several lines of evidence have implicated VP1 in the neutralization process. Regions of VP1, 2, and 3 are located on the capsid surface [8]. Cross-linking studies with neutralizing antipoliovirus antibody suggested recognition of one or more epitopes on VP1 [39]. Synthetic VP1 was reported to induce neutralizing antibodies [40,41]; in another study, synthetic oligopeptides from three regions on VP1 were found to prime or enhance the immune response of rabbits to subsequent exposure to whole poliovirus [42]. Minor and colleagues selected poliovirus type 3 substrains resistant to neutralizing monoclonal antibodies; by analyzing oligonucleotide abnormalities in these strains, they defined a major antigenic site on VP1 broadly between bases 277 and 294 [43,44]. While VP1 thus appears to be immunodominant in the generation of neutralizing antibodies, it is likely that polyclonal neutralizing antisera also recognize neutralizing sites on VP2 and VP3 [45]. The role of VP1 as a determinant of poliovirus binding and infectivity characteristics is further emphasized by the observation that the insertion of six amino acids in an exposed ten–amino acid loop of VP1 from Lansing type 2 poliovirus into the analogous region in the type 1 Mahoney strain produces a chimeric virus that is recognized by both type 1 and type 2 antipoliovirus antisera [46].

Surface proteins involved in poliovirus neutralization partially determine patterns of virulence of the virus. As an example, in mice an inoculation of 100 or fewer virions of the Lansing type 2 poliovirus produces fatal paralytic poliomyelitis, whereas considerably larger inocula of Mahoney type 1 polio are entirely benign. Variants of P2/Lansing resistant to neutralization by monoclonal antibodies to the critical exposed loop on VP1 frequently show altered neurovirulence as compared with parent virus; both biological modifications (non-neutralization, attenuation of virulence) result from mutations in the critical ten–amino acid region in the loop site on VP1 [13,47,48]. It is striking that in the aforementioned chimeric virus described by LaMonica and colleagues, the presence of only six critical Lansing strain amino acids in VP1 enables Mahoney type 1 poliovirus to produce paralytic infection in mouse brain [46]. These observations provide strong evidence that the biological behavior of poliovirus is importantly influenced by selected surface proteins. It is also likely that noncoding regions of the polioviral genome help determine neurovirulence of the virus. Thus, a single nucleic acid substitution in the 5' noncoding region of the RNA of the Sabin type 3 virus can attenuate virulence in both humans and mice, possibly by altering viral replication [49].

RELATION TO MOTOR NEURON DISEASE

The motor specificity of infection by poliovirus has prompted the speculation that this virus may be causally related to motor neuron disorders such as spinal muscular atrophy or amyotrophic lateral sclerosis. There is little data supporting this possibility. Investigations have included analysis of histocompatibility types; extensive culturing of cerebrospinal fluid, serum, and brain from patients; analysis of antipoliovirus antibody titers; and probing of affected tissues with cDNA to poliovirus both in solubilized preparations and in situ; all have failed to implicate poliovirus in the pathogenesis of motor neuron disease [50]. At least one group has failed to detect inhibition of cellular metabolism suggestive of poliovirus by extracts of brains of motor neuron disease patients [51]. While the older motor neuron disease literature includes references to "chronic poliomyelitis," this is a descriptive term; such cases inevitably lack virological or serological evidence of ongoing poliovirus infection.

FUTURE

One can envision several potential directions for future research in the virology of poliovirus. It is conceivable, for example, that recent advances in understanding of the relationship between viral proteins and virulence will produce new strategies for poliovirus vaccination. Improved understanding of the genetics of the virus may allow production of viruses with improved antigenicity and more stable attenuation. Chimeric viruses may be produced with the ability to provoke antibodies to all three serotypes of poliovirus [52]. It is possible that synthetic oligopeptides may be devised either as primary vaccines or as boosters. It is also conceivable that enhanced knowledge of the molecular biology of poliovirus will lead to specific therapies for active poliovirus infection [53]. Whereas this may be largely irrelevant in Western society, active polio-myelitis remains an important neurologic problem in other parts of the world. Thus, it may be possible to devise specific inhibitors for the polioviral replicase or the proteases such as that which cleaves e1-IF; the former would block viral replication while the latter would prevent host cell protein synthesis inhibition. Such agents might be useful for active infection with either poliovirus or related pathogens such as the rhinoviruses or Coxsackie virus. Such treatments might have extensive veterinary application (e.g., foot and mouth disease) and might even have merit on a trial basis in disorders suspected to be viral in origin. Finally, it remains likely that an improved understanding of the basis of the motor specificity of poliovirus will provide insight into unique biological prop-erties of motor neurons, regardless of whether the motor specificity of infection arises at the receptor level or at some step in polioviral replication subsequent to cell entry.

Acknowledgments

I wish to acknowledge the generous support of The Pierre L. de Bourgknecht A.L.S. Research Foundation and the Cecil B. Day Investment Company, Inc. Drs. J. Miller, D. Figlewicz, and R. Finberg kindly criticized the manuscript, which was typed by E. Thompson.

REFERENCES

1. McHenry LC Jr. Garrison's history of neurology. Springfield, Ill.: Charles C Thomas, 1969.
2. Medin O. En epidemi af infantil paralysi. Hygiea (Stockholm) 1890;52:657–68.
3. Landsteiner K, Popper E. Ubertragung der poliomyelitis acuta auf Affen. Z Immun Forsch 1908;2:377–90.
4. Flexner S, Lewis PA. The transmission of acute poliomyelitis to monkeys. JAMA 1909;53:1639.
5. Flexner S, Lewis PA. The transmission of epidemic poliomyelitis to monkeys: a further note. JAMA 1909;53:23.
6. Bodian D. Emerging concept of poliomyelitis infection. Science 1955;12:105–8.
7. Luria SE, Darnell JE Jr, Baltimore D, et al. General virology. New York: Wiley, 1978, pp 251–342.
8. Hogle JM, Chow M, Filman DJ. Three-dimensional structure of poliovirus at 2.9 A resolution. Science 1985;229:1358–65.
9. Kitamura N, Semler BL, Rothberg PG, et al. Primary structure, gene organization and polypeptide expression of poliovirus RNA. Nature 1981;291:547–53.
10. Racaniello VR, Baltimore D. Molecular cloning of poliovirus cDNA and deter-mination of the complete nucleotide sequence of the viral genome. Proc Natl Acad Sci USA 1981;78:4887–91.
11. Pelletier J, Kaplan G, Racaniello VR, et al. Translational efficiency of poliovirus mRNA: mapping inhibitory cis-acting elements within the 5′ noncoding region. J Virol 1988;62:2219–27.

12. Holland JJ. Receptor affinities as major determinants of enterovirus tissue tropism in humans. Virology 1964;15:312–26.
13. Jubelt B, Narayan O, Johnson RT. Pathogenesis of human poliovirus infection in mice. II. Age dependency of paralysis. J Neuropath Exp Med 1980;39:149–59.
14. Brown RH Jr, Johnson D, Ogonowski M, et al. Type 1 human poliovirus binds to human synaptosomes. Ann Neurol 1987;21:64–70.
15. Holland JJ, McLaren JC, Styverton JT. The mammalian cell virus relationship. IV. Infections of naturally insusceptible cells with enterovirus RNA. J Exp Med 1959;40:65–80.
16. Mendelsohn C, Johnson B, Lionetti KA, et al. Transformation of a human poliovirus receptor gene into mouse cells. Proc Natl Acad Sci USA 1986;83:7845–9.
17. Medrano L, Greene H. Picornavirus receptors and picornavirus multiplication in human-mouse hybrid cell lines. Virology 1973;54:515–24.
18. Miller DA, Miller OJ, Dev VG, et al. Human chromosome 19 carries a poliovirus receptor gene. Cell 1974;1:167–73.
19. Siddique T, McKinney R, Hung W, et al. The poliovirus sensitivity gene is on chromosome 19q12-q13.2. Genomics 1988;3:156–60.
20. Krah DL, Crowell RL. A solid-phase assay of solubilized HeLa cell membrane receptors for binding group B coxsackieviruses and polioviruses. Virology 1982; 118:148-56.
21. Crowell RL, Landa BJ, Siak J-S. Picornavirus receptors in pathogenesis. In: Lonberg-Holm K, Philipson L, eds. Receptors and recognition (series B, vol 8), virus receptors, part 2: animal viruses. New York: Chapman and Hall, 1981, pp 171–84.
22. Minor PD, Pipkin PA, Hockley D, et al. Monoclonal antibodies which block cellular receptors for polioviruses. Virus Res 1984;1:203–12.
23. Nobis P, Zibbire R, Meyer G, et al. Production of a monoclonal antibody against an epitope on HeLa cells that is the functional poliovirus binding site. J Gen Virol 1985;66:2563–9.
24. Shepley MP, Sherry B, Weiner HL. Monoclonal antibody identification of a 100-kda membrane protein in HeLa cells and human spinal cord involved in poliovirus attachment. Proc Natl Acad Sci USA 1988;85:7743–7.
25. Mendelsohn CL, Wimmer E, Racaniello VR. Cellular receptor for poliovirus: molecular cloning, nucleotide sequence, and expression of a new member of the immunoglobulin superfamily. Cell 1989;56:855–65.
26. Greve JM, Davis G, Meyer AM, et al. The major human rhinovirus receptor is ICAM-1. Cell 1989;56:839–47.
27. White JM, Littman DR. Viral receptors of the immunoglobulin superfamily. Cell 1989;56:725–8.
28. Staunton DE, Merluzzi VJ, Rothlein R, et al. A cell adhesion molecule, ICAM-1, is the major surface receptor for rhinoviruses. Cell 1989;56:849–53.
29. Abraham G, Colonno RJ. Many rhinovirus serotypes share the same cellular receptor. J Virol 1984;51:340–5.
30. Rossmann MG, Arnold E, Erickson JW, et al. Structure of a human common cold virus and functional relationship to other picornaviruses. Nature 1985;317:145–53.
31. Lonberg-Holm K. The effect of concanavalin A on the early events of infection by rhinovirus type 2 and poliovirus type 2. J Gen Virol 1975;28:313–27.
32. Madshus IH, Olsnes S, Sandvig K. Mechanism of entry into the cytosol of poliovirus type 1: requirement for low pH. J Cell Biol 1984;98:1194–200.
33. Sonenberg N. Regulation of translation by poliovirus. Adv Virus Res 1987;33:175–204.

34. Bienkowska-Szewczyk K, Ehrenfeld E. An internal 5'-noncoding region required for translation of poliovirus RNA in vitro. J Virol 1988;62:3068–72.
35. Pelletier J, Kaplan G, Racaniello VR, et al. Cap-independent translation of poliovirus mRNA is conferred by sequence elements within the 5' noncoding region. Mol Cell Biol 1988;8:1103–12.
36. Pelletier J, Sonenberg N. Internal initiation of translation of eukaryotic mRNA directed by a sequence derived from poliovirus RNA. Nature 1988;334:320–5.
37. Watson JD, Hopkins NH, Roberts JW, et al. Molecular biology of the gene, Vol II. Menlo Park, Calif: Benjamin-Cummings, 1987.
38. Chow M, Newman JFE, Filman D, et al. Myristylation of picornavirus capsid protein VP4 and its structural significance. 1987;327:482–6.
39. Emini EA, Jameson BA, Lewis AJ, et al. Poliovirus neutralization epitopes: analysis and localization with neutralizing monoclonal antibodies. J Virol 1982;43:997–1005.
40. Blondel B, Crainic R, Horodniceanu FC. R Hebd Seanc Acad Sci [Paris] 294:91–4.
41. Chow M, Baltimore D. Isolated poliovirus capsid protein VP1 induces a neutralizing response in rats. Proc Natl Acad Sci USA 1982;79:7518–21.
42. Emini EA, Jameson BA, Wimmer E. Priming for and induction of anti-poliovirus neutralizing antibodies by synthetic peptides. Nature 1983;304:699–703.
43. Evans DMA, Minor PD, Schild GS, et al. Critical role of an eight-amino acid sequence of VP1 in neutralization of poliovirus type 3. Nature 1983;304:459–62.
44. Minor PD, Schild GC, Bootman J, et al. Location and primary structure of a major antigenic site for poliovirus neutralization. Nature 1983;301:674–9.
45. Wimmer E, Jameson BA, Emini EA. Poliovirus antigenic sites and vaccines. Nature 1984;308:19.
46. Murray MG, Bradley J, Yang X-F, et al. Poliovirus host range is determined by a short amino acid sequence in neutralization antigenic site I. Science 1988;241:213–5.
47. LaMonica N, Almond JW, Racaniello VR. A mouse model for poliovirus neurovirulence identifies mutations that attenuate the virus for humans. J Virol 1987;61:2917–20.
48. LaMonica N, Kupsky WJ, Racaniello VR. Reduced mouse neurovirulence of poliovirus type 2 Lansing antigenic variants selected with monoclonal antibodies. Virology 1987;161:429–37.
49. Evans DMA, Dunn G, Minor PD, et al. Increased neurovirulence associated with a single nucleotide change in a noncoding region of the Sabin type 3 poliovirus genome. Nature 1983;314:548–50.
50. Brown RH Jr, Weiner HL. The relationship between poliovirus and amyotrophic lateral sclerosis. In: Rose FC, ed. Research progress in motor neurone disease. London: Pitman, 1984, pp 349–59.
51. Fallis RJ, Weiner LP. Further studies in search of a virus in amyotrophic lateral sclerosis. In: Rowland LP, ed. Human motorneuron diseases. New York: Raven, 1982, pp 355–61.
52. Burke KL, Dunn G, Ferguson M, et al. Antigen chimeras of poliovirus as potential new vaccines. Nature 1988;332:81–2.
53. Minor PD, Kew O, Schild GC. Poliomyelitis—epidemiology, molecular biology and immunology. Nature 1982;299:109–10.

Chapter 3

Post-Polio Syndrome: Definition of an Elusive Concept

Lauro S. Halstead

The concept of post-polio syndrome remains elusive for one principal reason: the level of our knowledge concerning the pathogenesis remains inadequate. With inadequate, incomplete, or inaccurate knowledge, our treatment modalities may be wrong or misguided and the taxonomy misleading. And without an accurate taxonomy, we are all a little like Kipling's blind Indians describing a different part of the elephant but unaware of the bigger reality. However, has this not been true for just about every disease in the history of medicine? In fact, the history of any individual disease is usually the story of progressing from the general to the specific as more information becomes available. Thus, the taxonomy of a disease is only as good as the knowledge base that underlies it.

Where we are exactly at the present time in our journey from complete ignorance to total understanding of late complications of polio is impossible to say. Nor is it possible to say what level of sophistication might be required to effect that understanding and a possible cure. However, it is clear that we have learned a great deal in recent years but not enough to propose definitive names much less definitive treatments. In the meantime, we must deal with what we have. In the rest of this chapter, I will briefly review some of the basic elements that have contributed to our current understanding of the elusive and rather recent concept of post-polio syndrome. These elements include (1) historic background, (2) epidemiologic aspects of the residual post-polio population in this country, (3) possible pathologic mechanisms for new health problems, (4) clinical features, (5) the clinical evaluations, (6) differential diagnosis, and (7) post-polio diagnoses and definitions.

HISTORICAL BACKGROUND

For more than 100 years, it has been recognized that there are late sequelae of polio that occur in some patients many years after their initial illness. The first descriptions appeared in 1875 when three patients were reported in the French literature [1–3]. All of the cases involved young men who had a history of paralytic polio in infancy and then, many years later as young adults, developed significant new weakness and atrophy. What is of particular interest in these cases is that the weakness and atrophy occurred not only in previously affected muscles but, in at least two instances, in previously unaffected muscles, also. In addition, all of the subjects had physically demanding jobs that required strength and repetitive activities. In a commentary on one of the cases [1], the great nineteenth-century French neuropathologist Jean Martin Charcot suggested several hypotheses for these new changes that are still relevant today. He believed that one spinal disorder made a patient more susceptible to a subsequent spinal disorder and that the new weakness was due to overuse of the involved limbs.

Since those initial reports there has only been sporadic interest in this phenomenon. In the century following Charcot's observations, there were less than thirty-five published reports that altogether described fewer than 250 cases [4]. As with the first subjects, these reports described new problems that included weakness, atrophy, and fasciculations occurring up to seventy-one years after an acute and generally severe attack of paralytic poliomyelitis. These neurological changes were most commonly diagnosed as a form of progressive muscular atrophy, although many other diagnostic terms were used, such as chronic anterior poliomyelitis, late motor neuron degeneration, and forme fruste amyotrophic lateral sclerosis [5–7].

Why the late sequelae of polio remained an obscure and largely unexplored corner of medicine until recently is not entirely clear. Few diseases are as widely prevalent in the world and have been as intensively investigated. Part of the explanation may lie in the fact that over the years polio has been viewed as a classic example of an acute viral infectious disease. Therefore, most of the energy and resources were directed at early management and prevention. Following widespread use of vaccines, polio quickly became a medical oddity in the industrialized world and interest and funding in polio-related problems waned. Part of the explanation may also lie in the fact that the big epidemics in this century did not occur until the 1940s and 1950s. Affected individuals are now thirty to forty years postonset, when new neurological changes tend to appear. Thus, many thousands of polio survivors are now experiencing new problems related to polio and by sheer weight of numbers are finally attracting attention among the medical and lay communities.

There are other reasons why the late sequelae have remained obscure and elusive. These include psychological, sociological, and even linguistic issues. To begin with, prior to 1980 the name did not exist and without a name it was not possible to talk or write about it. Even with a name, the concept or possibility of late sequelae of polio was not widely accepted or appreciated. Although there have been occasional reports in the literature to the contrary, the conventional wisdom in most medical and lay circles was that acute poliomyelitis resulted in a chronic, stable lesion. As late as 1982, polio was classified in a major rehabilitation text as an example of a static disease [8]. In addition, there was the knowledge that polio had been around for millennia and was one of the most widely prevalent and extensively studied diseases of all time. What else was there to learn? And worse, who cared? After all, polio was conquered, a disease of the past. The bright young minds had been attracted elsewhere and there was no scientific constituency to lobby for funds or research. The only people with a vested interest were the polio survivors themselves. But prior to 1980, they were isolated and fragmented. Their collective experience had not been tapped, and individually, if they were experiencing new symptoms, they tended to be discounted or misdiagnosed. A single patient with a "new" disease or syndrome is badly mismatched when confronted with the authority of a single physician who has not heard of an entity or, if so, does not believe that it exists.

EPIDEMIOLOGICAL ASPECTS

Accurate figures about the number of people who are experiencing new polio-related problems are not available currently and most likely will never be known. Data from the Household Survey of Disabling Conditions conducted by the National Center for Health Statistics in 1987 found that there were over 640,000 people who had experienced paralytic polio [9]. In the meantime, there has been an unknown amount of attrition from the polio population due to death since the 1987 survey. However, there has also been an unknown—and largely unexpected—increase in the number of polio survivors in this country resulting from the influx of affected immigrants, refugees, and illegal aliens who settled here over the past several decades from Southeast Asia and Latin America.

In 1984, a population-based study of residents in Rochester, Minnesota, by researchers at the Mayo Clinic, found that one in four people who had a history of paralytic polio were experiencing new problems probably related to their earlier illness. If the Mayo Clinic study is representative of the experience of polio survivors elsewhere in this country, then there are approximately 160,000 people in the United States who are currently experiencing new polio-related problems and may be in need of rehabilitation services. (An update of the Mayo Clinic study suggests that 160,000 may be low. A comprehensive follow-up evaluation of a random sample of the original respondents showed that 66% were experiencing new weakness [10].) However, regardless of the numbers experiencing new problems now, it is reasonable to assume that they will continue to increase as the post-polio population ages.

POSSIBLE PATHOLOGIC MECHANISMS

The pathologic changes that underlie the late complications of polio are incompletely understood. However, there are at least three processes that may play a role singly or in combination in any individual patient: (1) motor unit dysfunction, (2) musculoskeletal overuse, and (3) musculoskeletal disuse. Each may produce the cardinal symptom of progressive weakness. These three etiologic mechanisms and their associated complications and potential interactions are shown schematically in Figure 3.1. Thus far, the neurological or motor unit changes have attracted the most attention, but in the final analysis may not be any more prevalent or damaging than those caused by nonneurological changes. The pathologic mechanism of musculoskeletal disuse and the resultant complications of weakness, contractures, atrophy, diminished

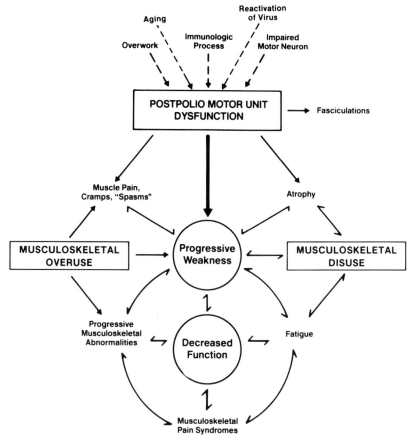

FIGURE 3.1   *Schematic model showing three possible causes for the late neuromuscular complications of polio and their interactions.*

endurance, and so forth are most likely similar to the disuse phenomenon that has been extensively studied and described in other groups of patients who have neuromuscular lesions and/or lead sedentary life-styles. The pathologic process of musculoskeletal overuse, on the other hand, is not as well understood. Evidence based on clinical and animal studies with a variety of lesions, including polio, suggests a relationship between muscle damage, the intensity of exercise, the number of motor units, and the duration of exercise [11]. Nonetheless, it is not known to what extent a primary muscle defect may be contributing to late onset weakness in some polio patients. However, regardless of the cause of weakness, many of these patients experience an overuse phenomenon from chronic mechanical strain on joints, ligaments, and soft tissues that have been improperly or inadequately supported for thirty or more years. The consequence of this overuse creates a self-perpetuating chain reaction of symptoms and further complications until effective interventions are implemented.

The cause of apparently new motor unit dysfunction in polio survivors many years after their acute illness is unknown. However, there are a number of theories, and evidence is accumulating to support several of these. One theory suggests that there may be persistence of the polio virus or viral fragments that have lain dormant and then are reactivated by some unknown trigger mechanism. Although it has been shown that polio virus can cause persistent asymptomatic infection in animals [12], this phenomenon has not been demonstrated in human studies as yet. Another theory suggests an immunological mechanism may be playing a role. Preliminary evidence to support this has been described by Dalakas et al., who found a lymphocytic response in muscle biopsies and immunoglobulin G (IgG) oligoclonal bands in the cerebrospinal fluid (CSF) of some symptomatic patients. By contrast, no oligoclonal bands were found in the CSF of a group of asymptomatic patients [13]. However, these findings have yet to be confirmed by other investigators, and patients generally have not responded to immunosuppressant therapy. A third possibility concerns changes in the spinal cord that might compromise motor neuron function. A recent report by Pezeshkpour and Dalakas described active inflammatory gliosis, neuronal chromatolysis, and axonal spheroids in the spinal cords of polio patients who died many years later of other causes. Whether these changes represent a primary lesion in the cord or a response to a lesion in the distal axon is unknown [14].

Another hypothesis is that the new neuromuscular changes are caused by premature aging of the polio patient. In normal individuals, significant attrition of motor neurons does not occur until the seventh decade [15]. However, in polio survivors with a greatly reduced population of anterior horn cells, the loss of relatively few giant motor units might result in a disproportionate loss of clinical function. While this hypothesis is intuitively attractive and may, in fact, explain new weakness in some individuals, muscle biopsy studies for the most part have failed to show significant group atrophy and other changes that would be consistent with new loss of whole motor units. Further, if motor neuron loss with advancing age were a major factor, then one would expect to find a steady increase in new difficulties as the population at risk became progressively older. In fact, several studies have failed to show a positive relationship between the onset of new weakness and chronological age [10,16]. To the contrary, these studies suggest that it is the *length* of the interval between onset of polio and the appearance of new symptoms that is a determining variable.

Finally, a fifth theory, and the most plausible in light of the limited information available at this time, suggests that the new clinical changes are a result of motor neuron overwork that eventually produces neuronal dysfunction. This theory is based on several assumptions and observations. The giant motor units that are characteristic of post-polio reinnervated muscles create an increased metabolic demand on the remaining motor neurons. The increased metabolic load, this theory states, eventually results in neurological dysfunction after a critical number of years. This concept of overuse is supported indirectly by several clinical studies and electromyographic (EMG) data. In a group of seventeen patients evaluated in a post-polio clinic, Maynard observed that new weakness occurred more commonly in the legs than in the arms [17]. Similarly, in the Mayo Clinic study, Windebank and co-workers found that in muscles with similar involvement at onset of polio, new weakness occurred more commonly in the weightbearing muscles of the legs than in the nonweight-bearing muscles of the arms. Further, new weakness was more likely to occur in limbs most affected by the original disease [10]. In another study, Perry et al. observed that in subjects with approximately the same residual loss, symptomatic polio survivors had a less efficient gait with an increase in intensity as well as duration of contraction of extensor muscles in the legs when compared with asymptomatic polio survivors [18].

Electrophysiological studies by Wiechers, Dalakas, and others have shown neuromuscular transmission abnormalities that suggest that the giant motor neurons may not be able to sustain indefinitely the metabolic demands of all their sprouts, resulting in a slow deterioration of individual terminals and a drop-off of reinnervated muscle fibers [13,19]. As more muscle fibers are lost, slowly progressive weakness becomes clinically apparent. Figure 3.2 shows an increase in jitter and blocking on single-fiber EMG with increased time after polio in a group of asymptomatic subjects, which is consistent with the theory of a gradual deterioration of individual peripheral nerve terminals. These observations are in contrast to static nerve injuries where electrophysiological stability is achieved after reinnervation within a period of twelve to eighteen months.

Related to the overwork theory is the possibility that the original viral attack on the anterior horn cells left some motor neurons functional but impaired, and thus more vulnerable to dysfunction with the passage of time. Tomlinson noted in the spinal cords of persons surviving long after the polio attack that many of the neurons are smaller than normal in size. Based on this observation and the work of Bodian, he concluded that any cell invaded by

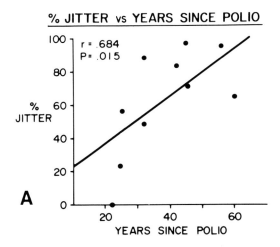

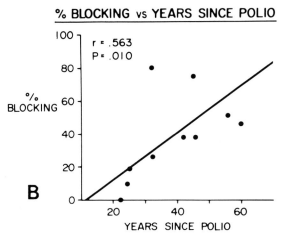

FIGURE 3.2 (A) *Relationship between the percentage of motor unit recordings with abnormal jitter found in each patient with polio and the number of years elapsed since the attack of polio. Analysis by product-moment correlation and rank-order correlation coefficients showed a significant association (r = 0.684, p = 0.05) between the percentage of jitter found and the number of years since the attack of polio. (B) Relationship between the percentage of motor unit recordings demonstrating blocking found in each patient with polio and the number of years elapsed since the attack of polio. Analysis by product-moment correlation and rank-order correlation coefficients showed a significant association (r = 0.563, p = 0.010) between the percentage of blocking and the number of years since the attack of polio. (Reprinted with permission from Wiechers et al. [19].)*

the polio virus is likely to be permanently affected, particularly in relation to "protein synthetic mechanisms" [20]. Thus, it seems possible that some motor neurons experienced an injury at the time of the acute infection that is then exacerbated by many years of increased metabolic demand to sustain a greatly enlarged motor unit.

CLINICAL FEATURES

In response to the increased recognition of new health problems in the polio population, a number of post-polio clinics have opened in various parts of the country over the past few years. The observations reported by these clinics and in a number of research studies have helped clarify the major clinical features presented by post-polio patients. The experience obtained in the Post-Polio Clinic at the Institute for Rehabilitation and Research in Houston, Texas, is fairly typical and is summarized in Tables 3.1 and 3.2. Table 3.1 lists the most common new health and functional problems in 132 consecutive people seen over a one-year period. All patients were carefully evaluated to confirm the diagnosis of old polio and rule out nonpolio causes for their new symptoms. The majority of patients were women (66%), white (92%), and middle-aged (median age forty-five years, with a range from twenty-four to eighty-six years). In addition, most were married, well educated, working outside the home, and

Table 3.1   Most Common New Health and Functional Problems for 132 Consecutive Patients with Confirmed Polio

	N	%
Health problems		
Fatigue	117	89
Muscle pain	93	71
Joint pain	93	71
Weakness		
Previously affected muscles	91	69
Previously unaffected muscles	66	50
Cold intolerance	38	29
Atrophy	37	28
Cramps	24	18
Fasciculations	16	12
ADL problems[a]		
Walking	84	64
Climbing stairs	80	61
Dressing	23	17

Note: Reprinted with permission from Halstead, et al. [16].
[a]ADL = activities of daily living.

Table 3.2   Number of Problems and Frequency of Persons Experiencing Each New Problem for the Six Most Common Problem Areas for 132 Post-Polio Patients

No. of Problems	No. of Persons	(%)	New Health Problems[a]					
			F	*P*	*W*	*FL*	*CI*	*A*
2	11	(8)	4	7	4	3	2	0
3	22	(17)	17	15	14	11	1	2
4	51	(39)	48	46	45	45	4	7
5	36	(27)	33	32	33	32	18	16
6	12	(9)	12	12	12	12	12	12
Total	132	(100)	117	113	110	103	38	37

Note: Reprinted with permission from Halstead et al. [16].
[a]F = fatigue; P = pain in muscles and/or joints; W = weakness in previously affected and/or unaffected muscles; FL = functional loss in walking, climbing stairs, dressing, and so forth; CI = cold intolerance; A = new atrophy.

about thirty-five to forty years postonset of acute polio. The median age at onset of polio was seven years (range three months to forty-four years) with a median interval between onset of polio and onset of new health problems of thirty-one years. This interval is similar to that found in other studies, but the range has been reported to extend from two to eight decades [13,16].

In general, it has been found that patients most at risk for developing new problems are those who experienced more severe polio at onset, although it is not unusual to see patients with typical post-polio symptoms who had seemingly very mild polio with excellent clinical recovery. In addition to severity at onset, the age at onset is associated with the development of late onset problems. Thus, people who were older when they contracted polio appear to be at an increased risk for experiencing new neurological symptoms. Most commonly, the onset of these new problems is insidious, but in many people they may be precipitated by specific events such as a minor accident, fall, period of bedrest, or weight gain. Characteristically, patients state that a similar event experienced several years earlier would not have caused the same decline in health and function. Likewise, new problems may begin when coexisting medical problems, such as diabetes, develop or worsen.

While the frequency distribution of the problems listed in Table 3.1 may differ from clinic to clinic, it is increasingly clear that there is a common set of complaints that is quite specific to the post-polio patient. Further, as shown in Table 3.2, there is often a cluster of problems that occur together. In the Houston patients, the most common cluster (experienced by 39%) consisted of excessive fatigue, pain, weakness, and functional loss. New atrophy was relatively uncommon (28%); when it was present, it did not occur as an isolated finding but tended to be present when there were four or more other problems.

Clinical Evaluation

Because of the number and diversity of problems frequently presented by post-polio patients, an interdisciplinary evaluation by several professionals is desirable, if possible. In addition to the physician, we have found it helpful to include a physical therapist, occupational therapist, orthotist, and social worker as part of the initial evaluation team with referral to other disciplines and medical specialists as needed. Because post-polio–related complications are diagnosed by exclusion, it is essential that every patient receive a careful history and physical exam, along with appropriate laboratory studies, radiographs, and diagnostic tests to rule out other medical, orthopedic, or neurological conditions that might be causing or aggravating the presenting symptoms. Regardless of the underlying etiology, however, a psychosocial evaluation is invariably helpful, together with an assessment of function, gait, orthotic needs, and a baseline measure of strength and endurance of key muscle groups. For most patients, an EMG and nerve conduction velocity (EMG/NCV) is useful to help confirm the presence of prior polio, identify possible subclinical involvement, establish a baseline, and help exclude other neurological conditions. However, a standard battery of screening tests, such as an SMA 24, thyroid panel, Tensilon test, and so forth, used on a routine basis is generally not helpful or cost effective. Some clinicians monitor creatinine phosphokinase on a regular basis, but the diagnostic and clinical implications, if any, are still not clear. Patients who had respiratory involvement initially and have a history of pulmonary disease should have pulmonary function studies and, if indicated, arterial blood gases.

Finally, all attempts to find laboratory tests or diagnostic studies that distinguish the symptomatic from the asymptomatic post-polio so far have been unsuccessful. Furthermore, there is still no objective method to predict who might become symptomatic in the future or to monitor the progress of the underlying pathology in the subject who has already become symptomatic. Specifically, no serological, enzymatic, or electrodiagnostic test has been helpful to separate the symptomatic from the asymptomatic groups. Unfortunately, these negative findings have contributed to the elusive quality of a post-polio diagnosis and skepticism in some minds. And yet, most of the researchers and clinicians who have worked with polio survivors—to say nothing of the thousands of people who are experiencing new symptoms—are convinced that a post-polio clinical entity does in fact exist.

Differential Diagnosis

There are three major criteria that should be established to make a diagnosis of a polio-related problem: (1) objective evidence of a prior episode of paralytic polio; (2) a characteristic pattern of recovery and neurological stability preceding the onset of new problems; and (3) exclusion of other medical, orthopedic, and neurological conditions that might cause the presenting symptoms.

The first two criteria are usually easier to satisfy than the third. The diagnosis of paralytic polio can almost always be confirmed with the following information: (1) a credible history of an acute, febrile illness resulting in motor loss and no sensory loss; (2) the occurrence of a similar illness in family or neighborhood contacts; (3) the presence of focal, asymmetric weakness and/or atrophy on examination; (4) changes on EMG of chronic denervation compatible with prior anterior horn cell disease; and (5) examination of the original medical records whenever possible. The changes on routine EMG compatible with prior polio include increased amplitude and duration of motor unit action potentials, an increase in the percentage of polyphasic motor units, and a decrease in the number of motor units on maximum recruitment. Occasionally, positive sharp waves and fibrillations are present and, less commonly, fasciculations may be seen.

In patients with late complications of polio, the pattern of events from onset of polio to onset of new problems is so characteristic that when it is absent the diagnosis should be seriously questioned. The pattern generally consists of four stages as shown in Figure 3.3: (1) paralytic polio in childhood or later in life; (2) partial to fairly complete neurological and functional recovery; (3) a period of functional and neurological stability lasting many years, usually twenty or more; and (4) the gradual or abrupt onset of one or more of the new health problems listed in Table 3.1. Most students of post-polio agree that one of the new problems should include *nondisuse weakness*. However, for practical reasons, nondisuse weakness may be difficult to docu-

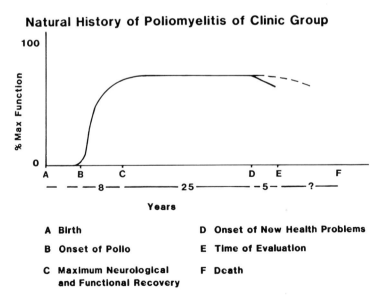

FIGURE 3.3 *Functional changes at key milestones for 132 persons with post-polio syndrome (solid line). Note interval D–E is five years.*

ment, although it frequently can be inferred by the onset of diminished function despite maintaining the usual level and intensity of activity.

There are several dilemmas in making a polio-related diagnosis in this population: (1) the symptoms are frequently so general that ruling out all possible causes is not practical and can be prohibitively expensive; (2) there is no direct evidence for a causal relation between the earlier polio and the new neurologic changes; (3) there are no definitive tests; (4) the diagnosis is one of exclusion; and (5) coexisting medical, orthopedic, and/or neurological conditions may be present that can produce a similar set of overlapping signs and symptoms, as shown in Figure 3.4. Examples of such conditions include compression neuropathies, radiculopathies, degenerative arthritis, disc disease, obesity, anemia, diabetes, thyroid disease, depression, and so forth. In addition, as indicated in Figure 3.1, once a problem, such as weakness, occurs—regardless of the underlying etiology—it may initiate a chain reaction of other complications that makes the original problem impossible to identify. Nonetheless, because of the central importance of new weakness in this population and because of its diagnostic and management implications, every effort should be made to exclude disuse weakness as a major factor.

Likewise, the role of chronic musculoskeletal wear and tear should be clarified. Many of the problems that appear to be related to overuse of weakened muscles as well as abnormal joint and limb biomechanics may simply represent the normal consequences of chronic disability and be no more common in post-polios than they are in individuals with other neuromuscular diseases. In any event, the management of overuse complications is fairly straightforward. Most people respond favorably to conservative interventions aimed at reducing mechanical stress, supporting weakened muscles, and stabilizing abnormal joint movements. If chronic overuse is the only or major

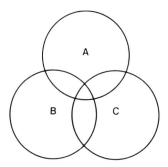

A = Signs and Symptoms of Neurologic Dysfunction
B = Signs and Symptoms of Orthopedic Dysfunction
C = Signs and Symptoms of Non-Polio Medical Dysfunction

FIGURE 3.4   *Representation of possible combination of presenting complaints and their causes found in post-polio patients.*

underlying pathology present, then such interventions can often slow or prevent further deterioration and possibly lead to a reversal of symptoms and improved function.

Finally, every polio patient who presents with new symptoms should be carefully evaluated to exclude amyotrophic lateral sclerosis (ALS). Although there are often a number of similarities, there are enough dissimilarities that the two can usually be distinguished without great difficulty. Table 3.3 summarizes the major differential features found on clinical and laboratory exams. Over the years, there has been considerable speculation that an antecedent infection with polio might be associated with developing ALS later in life [21–23]. However, with the recent interest in the late complications of polio and the new understanding about some of the possible pathophysiologic mechanisms, it now seems likely that many of the patients who had polio and later were diagnosed as having a benign form of ALS were misdiagnosed. In a recent re-examination of five patients with a history of both polio and ALS, Brown and Patten concluded that none of the patients would now be classified as ALS but rather as post-polio syndrome [24].

POST-POLIO DIAGNOSES AND DEFINITIONS

Given the nonspecific nature of the symptoms and the absence of any definitive or pathognomonic tests, it is understandable why there is no clear consensus to date about the most appropriate names or diagnostic labels to use in post-polio patients with new health problems. A number of terms have been proposed, including post-polio syndrome, post-polio muscular atrophy, late effects of polio, and post-polio sequelae. One of the reasons that none of these terms is suitable for all individuals is the lack of specificity in diagnostic criteria. This, in turn, is related to our incomplete understanding of the underlying pathophysiology of the presenting complaints. Another reason no single term is suitable for all individuals is that there may be one, two, or more pathologic processes present at any one time producing similar, overlapping symptoms (Figures 3.1 and 3.4). Separating out the origin of each symptom may not only be impractical but impossible, which gives rise to the need for a more general and less precise diagnostic term.

At the present time, post-polio progressive muscular atrophy (PPMA) has the most specific criteria. This term applies to those patients who have documented objective evidence of neuromuscular deterioration and have had a muscle biopsy that shows evidence of active denervation in the form of scattered angulated fibers [13]. Based on the inconsistent presence of new atrophy in Dalakas' series and the growing body of evidence that suggests that motor neuron dysfunction may be manifested in many ways, we propose an alternative term to PPMA, namely, post-polio motor neuron disease (PMND). This new term has the advantage of being more generic, less restrictive, and possibly less misleading by de-emphasizing new atrophy.

Table 3.3 Comparison of Clinical and Laboratory Findings in Patients with Late Polio and Amyotrophic Lateral Sclerosis

Patients	Weakness	Bulbar Sxs	Fasciculations	Long Tract Signs	Sensory Changes	Prognosis
			Clinical Findings			
ALS	Often symmetrical, generalized	Common	Common	Very common	Absent	Rapid downhill course; death 3–5 yr.
Post-polio	Asymmetrical focal	Rare	Occasional	Very rare	Absent	Slow progression 1%/yr.

Patients	DNA Repair	CPK	EMG	Muscle Biopsy
		Laboratory Findings		
ALS	Abnormal	Frequently elevated	Fibrillations and PSW[a] +++; fasciculations +++; MUP-rarely > 10 mV; fiber density jitter/blocking ↑↑; neurogenic jitter ↑↑, often present	Group atrophy common; scattered angulated fibers; inflammation rare
Post-polio	Normal	Occasionally elevated	Fibrillations and PSW +; fasciculations +; MUP-often > 10 mV; fiber density ↑↑; jitter/blocking ↑↑; neurogenic jitter rare	Group atrophy uncommon; inflammation in 40%

Note: Adapted with permission from Dalakas MC. Amyotrophic lateral sclerosis and post-polio: differences and similarities. In: Halstead LS, Wiechers DO, eds. Research and clinical aspects of the late effects of poliomyelitis. White Plains, NY: March of Dimes, 1987.
[a]PSW = positive sharp waves; MUP = motor unit potential.

Table 3.4 Criteria for the Diagnosis of Post-Polio Syndrome

A prior episode of paralytic polio confirmed by history, physical exam, and EMG.

A period of neurologic recovery followed by an extended interval of functional stability preceding the onset of new problems. The interval of neurologic and functional stability usually lasts 20 or more years.

The gradual or abrupt onset of non-disuse weakness in previously affected and/or unaffected muscles. This may or may not be accompanied by other new health problems, such as excessive fatigue, muscle pain, joint pain, decreased endurance, decreased function, atrophy, and so forth.

Standard EMG evaluation demonstrates changes consistent with prior AHC disease; fibrillations, sharp waves, and increased percent of polyplastic potentials may or may not be present.

Exclusion of medical, orthopedic, and neurologic conditions that might cause the health problems listed earlier.

In contrast to PPMA (or PMND), post-polio syndrome is a more heterogeneous term and therefore more practical in the typical clinical setting. However, it should not be used indiscriminately for every person with a history of paralytic polio with a new complaint. Criteria for making this diagnosis are outlined in Table 3.4. These criteria are based on the assumption that the pathologic process involves some motor unit dysfunction with a variable contribution from musculoskeletal overuse. For this reason, the presence of non-disuse weakness is considered a necessary finding to make this diagnosis. Ideally, then, the diagnosis of post-polio syndrome should only be made after a trial of closely supervised exercise to exclude the possibility of disuse weakness. As new information becomes available about the underlying mechanisms that produce late onset complications, these criteria will undoubtedly change and new terminology will be developed to fit our improved understanding.

REFERENCES

1. Raymond M (with contribution by Charcot JM). Paralysie essentiele de l'énfance: atrophie musculaire consecutive. Gaz Med [Paris] 1875;225.
2. Cornil L. Sur un cas de paralysie generale spinale anterieure subaigue, suivi d'autopsie. Gaz Med [Paris] 1875;4:127–9.
3. Carriere. Amytrophies secondaire. These de Montpelier, 1875.
4. Wiechers DO. Late effects of polio: historical perspectives. In: Halstead LS, Wiechers DO, eds. Research and clinical aspects of the late effects of poliomyelitis. White Plains, NY: March of Dimes, 1987, pp 1–12.

5. Kayser-Gatchalian MC. Late muscular atrophy after poliomyelitis. Eur Neurol 1973;10:371–80.
6. Campbell AMG, Williams ER, Pearce J. Late motor neuron degeneration following poliomyelitis. Neurology [Minneapolis] 1969;19:1101–6.
7. Mulder DW, Rosenbaum RA, Layton DD. Late progression of poliomyelitis or forme fruste amyotrophic lateral sclerosis? Mayo Clin Proc 1972;47:756–61.
8. Johnson EW, Alexander MA. Management of motor unit diseases. In: Kottke FJ, Stilwell GK, Lehmann JF, eds. Krusen's handbook of physical medicine and rehabilitation, ed 3. Philadelphia: WB Saunders, 1982, pp 679–90.
9. National Health Survey. Prevalence of selected impairments (series 10) Washington, DC: U.S. Department of Health and Human Services (in press).
10. Windebank AJ, Daube JR, Litchy WJ, et al. Late sequelae of paralytic poliomyelitis in Olmstead County, Minnesota. In: Halstead LS, Wiechers DO, eds. Research and clinical aspects of the late effects of poliomyelitis. White Plains, NY: March of Dimes, 1987, pp 27–38.
11. Herbison GJ, Jaweed MM, Ditunno JF. Exercise therapies in peripheral neuropathies. Arch Phys Med Rehabil 1983;64:201–5.
12. Miller JR. Prolonged intracerebral infection with poliomyelitis in asymptomatic mice. Ann Neurol 1981;9:590–6.
13. Dalakas MC, Elder G, Hallett M, et al. A long-term follow-up study of patients with post-poliomyelitis neuromuscular symptoms. N Engl J Med 1986;314:959–63.
14. Pezeshkpour GH, Dalakas MC. Pathology of spinal cord in postpoliomyelitis muscular atrophy. In: Halstead LS, Wiechers DO, eds. Research and clinical aspects of the late effects of poliomyelitis. White Plains, NY: March of Dimes, 1987, pp 229–36.
15. Tomlinson BE, Irving D. The numbers of limb motor neurons in the human lumbosacral cord throughout life. J Neurol Sci 1977;34:213–9.
16. Halstead LS. Late effects of polio: clinical experience with 132 consecutive outpatients. In: Halstead LS, Wiechers DO, eds. Research and clinical aspects of the late effects of poliomyelitis. White Plains, NY: March of Dimes, 1987, pp 13–26.
17. Maynard FM. Differential diagnosis of pain and weakness in post-polio patients. In: Halstead LS, Wierchers DO, eds. Late effects of poliomyelitis. Miami: Symposia Foundation, 1985, pp 33–44.
18. Perry J, Barnes G, Granley JK. Post polio muscle function. In: Halstead LS, Wiechers DO, eds. Research and clinical aspects of the late effects of poliomyelitis. White Plains, NY: March of Dimes, 1987, pp 315–28.
19. Wiechers DO, Hubbell SL. Late changes in the motor unit after acute poliomyelitis. Muscle Nerve 1981;4:524–8.
20. Tomlinson BE, Irving D. Changes in spinal cord motor neurons of possible relevance to the late effects of poliomyelitis. In: Halstead LS, Wiechers DO, eds. Late effects of poliomyelitis. Miami: Symposia Foundation, 1985, pp 57–72.
21. Poskanzer DC, Cantor HM, Kaplan GS. The frequency of preceding poliomyelitis in amyotrophic lateral sclerosis. In: Norris FH Jr, Kurland LT, eds. Motor neuron diseases: research on amyotrophic lateral sclerosis and related disorders. New York: Grune & Stratton, 1969, pp 286–90.
22. Pierce-Ruhland R, Patten BM. Repeat study of antecedent events in motor neuron disease. Ann Clin Res 1981;13:102–7.
23. Zilkha KJ. Untitled discussion. Proc R Soc Med 1962;55:1028–9.
24. Brown S, Patten BM. Post-polio syndrome and amyotrophic lateral sclerosis: a relationship more apparent than real. In: Halstead LS, Wiechers DO, eds. Research and clinical aspects of the late effects of poliomyelitis. White Plains, NY: March of Dimes, 1987, pp 83–98.

Chapter 4

Post-Polio Syndrome: Clues from Muscle and Spinal Cord Studies

Marinos Dalakas

Before discussing the pathogenesis of post-polio syndrome based on clues derived from our histological studies on muscle and spinal cords, it is pertinent to discuss the spectrum of the clinical symptomatology as it relates to the histopathological findings. We define post-polio syndrome as including the new neuromuscular symptoms that some patients develop twenty-five to thirty-five years after reaching maximum recovery from acute paralytic poliomyelitis [1–9]. These symptoms are unrelated to any other neurologic, orthopedic, psychiatric, or systemic medical illnesses and include the following:

- *Musculoskeletal complaints,* the indirect result of the late effects of polio, such as joint pains, fatigue, decreased physical endurance, back pain, and early symptoms of "wear and tear" in biomechanically disadvantaged joints.
- *Post-poliomyelitis progressive muscular atrophy (PPMA),* which describes new muscle weakness affecting certain muscle groups (including rarely the bulbar and respiratory muscles) with or without muscular atrophy or pain [1–9].

The summary of the clinical symptoms and signs of patients with post-polio syndrome that we have included in our study and described previously in detail [1–9], are summarized in Table 4.1. The inclusive criteria satisfied by our studied patients [9] are summarized in Table 4.2.

Motor neurons are the direct primary target of the poliomyelitis virus. As a result, the muscles supplied by the affected neurons show pathological changes that reflect the degree of the motor neuron damage and subsequent recovery. We have studied the morphology of muscle [9–14] and spinal cord [9,15,16] and we have performed electrophysiological studies in post-polio patients with a variety of symptoms, including those with predominantly musculoskeletal

Table 4.1   Symptoms and Signs of a Patient with Post-Polio Syndrome

---

Musculoskeletal
    Fatigue
    Decreased endurance
    Progressive increase in skeletal deformities (i.e., scoliosis or unusual body
        mechanics causing further deterioration of functional capacity)
    Pain in biomechanically disadvantaged, deformed, or marginally stable joints
New muscle weakness, the Progressive Post-poliomyelitis Muscular Atrophy (PPMA)
    New muscle weakness affecting muscles originally affected or spared
    New muscular atrophy
    Occasional pain and fasciculations in newly symptomatic or even asymptomatic
        muscles
    New bulbar, respiratory, or sleep difficulties, only in patients with residual bulbar
        and respiratory muscle weakness
A combination of musculoskeletal symptoms and PPMA

---

symptoms, patients with PPMA, and asymptomatic post-polio volunteers [6,9,17] in an attempt to make meaningful conclusions regarding the pathogenesis of the new symptomatology. Because development of post-polio symptoms relates directly to the recovery process after acute polio and the extent or severity of the original illness [6,9,18], the clinicopathological and electrophysiological aspects of the acute poliomyelitis will be reviewed first with emphasis on the morphology of the spinal cord, muscle, and motor nerve terminals.

CLINICOPATHOLOGIC FEATURES OF ACUTE POLIOMYELITIS

Spinal Cord

The pathological characteristics in the spinal cord of both acute human and experimental poliomyelitis infection have been described by Bodian [19–22].

Table 4.2   Diagnostic Criteria of Post-Polio Syndrome

---

1. History of an acute febrile paralytic illness during a polio epidemic with
   functional stability of recovery for at least 15 years
2. Residual, asymmetric muscle atrophy, weakness, and areflexia in at least one
   limb with normal sensation
3. Development of new neuromuscular symptoms
   Musculoskeletal complaints
   Progressive post-poliomyelitis muscular atrophy   (PPMA)
   Combination of the above two
4. Exclusion of back injuries, radiculopathies, compression neuropathies, and any
   other medical, neurologic, orthopedic, or psychiatric illness that could explain the
   symptoms mentioned above

A summary of the successive changes of the anterior horn cells after invasion by the polio virus based on Bodian's studies, appears in Table 4.3. The fate of an anterior horn cell attacked by poliovirus is shown in Figure 4.1. The following points in the spinal cord pathological evolution of acute poliomyelitis may bear on the pathogenesis of its late complications.

1. Acutely, the polio virus is not limited to motor neurons but it is universally disseminated within the central nervous system (CNS) (Table 4.4). Even in cases with circumscribed clinical symptoms, the pathologic abnormalities characteristically extend to other vulnerable regions of the CNS without

Table 4.3 Summary of the Most Pertinent Pathologic Changes in the Anterior Horn Cells of Successive Clinical Stages of Acute Paralytic Poliomyelitis

Preparalytic period
　　Diffuse thinning of basophilic substance of the neuron with complete dissolution in the late preparalytic stage
　　Formation of acidophilic nuclear inclusion bodies

First day of paralysis
　　Diffuse chromatolysis of motor neurons, necrosis, and neuronophagia
　　Few nuclear changes except if severe chromatolysis

Second and third days
　　Striking scarcity of normal-appearing neurons, even in cases of very mild paralysis[a]
　　Rapid changes with most of the destroyed neurons completely absorbed

Fourth to sixth days
　　Remarkable for the presence of only few normal neurons left, even with little functional loss
　　Very minimal, if any, active neuronophagia or necrosis present; surviving cells most likely would recover
　　Central chromatolysis begins, intermixed with neurons showing diffuse chromatolysis

Seventh to tenth days
　　Central chromatolysis predominates with intranuclear acidophilic inclusions
　　Greater proportion of normal or almost normal neurons are found

Third week
　　Rapid signs of recovery
　　Most of the cells are either normal in appearance (less than 10% being abnormal) or destroyed and removed
　　Very few irreversibly damaged—necrotic—cells are present
　　Central chromatolysis with signs of recovery of basophilic substance

Convalescent stage
　　Morphologic recovery of over 90% of surviving neurons by the first month
　　Disappearance of leukocytic infiltrates coinciding with the recovery of the remaining neurons
　　Perivascular cuffs markedly reduced by the sixth month, could persist up to one year
　　Gliosis

[a]This indicates the wide dissemination of the virus and supports the fact that many cells that are invaded by the virus later recover.

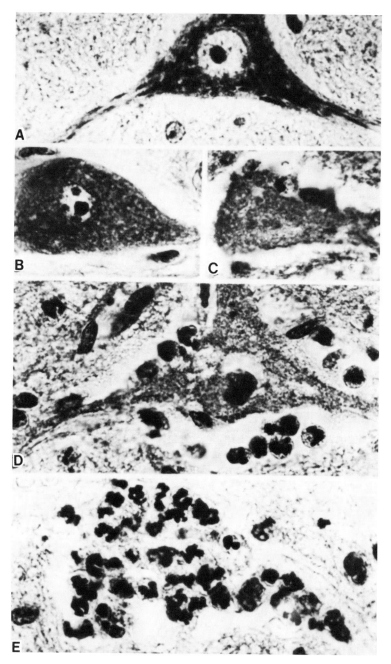

FIGURE 4.1 *Successive stages in destruction of an anterior horn cell of monkeys experimentally infected with poliovirus. (A) Normal neuron three days before onset of paralysis. (B) Diffuse chromatolysis and three acidophilic intranuclear inclusions grouped around the larger nucleus found almost exclusively in monkeys sacrificed one day before onset of paralysis. (C) Complete acidophilic necrosis. (D) Polymorphonuclear lymphocytes invading necrotic neuron. (E) Neuronophagia seen during the first day of paralysis. (Courtesy of Dr. A. Sabin.)*

Table 4.4 Distribution of Pathologic Changes within the Central Nervous System

Spinal cord
    Motor neurons of the anterior horn cells
    Neurons in the intermediate, intermediolateral, and posterior horns
    Dorsal root ganglia

Cortical neurons
    Precentral motor cortex, especially area 4 of Broadman
    Hypothalamus
    Globus pallidus

Cerebellum
    Cerebellar roof nuclei and vermis

Brainstem
    Nucleus ambiguous
    Facial, hypoglossal, vestibulbar, and trigeminal nuclei
    Reticular formation in medulla, pons, and midbrain

causing clinical abnormalities. The pathological changes, as summarized in Table 4.3, extend to the motor neurons of the anterior horn cells, especially the lumbosacral and cervical enlargement of the spinal cord, sparing the white matter. Cells in the intermediate, intermediolateral, and posterior horns often are affected and lesions commonly extend into the dorsal root ganglia. The hypothalamus, thalamus, precentral motor cortex, and at times the cerebellar roof nuclei and cerebellar vermis can be involved. The disease can affect several brain stem motor nuclear groups (bulbar poliomyelitis), including the nucleus ambiguous, facial, hypoglossal, and at times the trigeminal motor nuclei. Involvement of the reticular formation in the medulla, pons, and midbrain can cause ventilatory failure and central cardiorespiratory dysfunction. Permanent severe paralysis of the bulbar muscles is less common among survivors, probably because of the relatively small size of the motor units served by the brain stem nuclei [23].

2.   In regions related to acute paralysis, only 3 to 4% of neurons still appear normal two to five days after onset of paralysis. Furthermore, even in clinically unaffected or minimally affected segments of spinal cord, only about 10% of motor neurons look normal. During convalescence, the number of remaining neurons that look normal increases to almost 50% by one month [19–22].

3.   The proportion of destroyed motor neurons during the first week of acute paralysis is about 47% (based on the grand average of 120 limb populations examined by Bodian during this period) [19–22]. Since all but about 4% of motor neurons are involved in the acute stage, Bodian concluded that the average proportion of injured nerve cells that are destroyed, the "case fatality rate," is almost 50%, with a 30% probability that an invaded motor neuron would be destroyed by viral activity.

4.   Infected motor neurons exhibiting only mild degrees of diffuse chromatolysis most likely survive. The loss of function in muscle groups appears to correlate only with severe cytoplasmic and nuclear changes [19–22].

These observations of the pathologic changes may explain some of the mechanisms of new weakness in post-polio cases. Since every muscle is innervated by motor neurons from two to three contiguous levels of the spinal cord, even extensive destruction of the anterior horn cells limited to one level may not be expressed clinically in paralysis. This is evident in Figure 4.2 of a spinal cord from a rapidly fatal human case of bulbar poliomyelitis. Normal motor neurons without inflammation are noted at one level of the lumbar cord, whereas foci of neuronophagia and perivascular inflammation in the midst of normal neurons are seen at a contiguous level. Similar effects apply in animals that recover completely from mild paralysis as depicted in Figure 4.3, which shows spinal cord motor neurons of a monkey that has recovered from an acute paralytic attack.

In 90 to 95% of patients who survive severe poliomyelitis, the paralysis remains fixed for a period of days or weeks, after which improvement slowly follows. Sixty percent of eventual recovery is achieved by three months and 80% by six months. Minimal further improvement may continue over eighteen months to two years, possibly due in part to learning more effective use of weakened muscles or a delay in the recovery of some motor neurons with slow onset of terminal axon sprouting that takes longer to provide normal neuromuscular transmission to all reinnervated fibers.

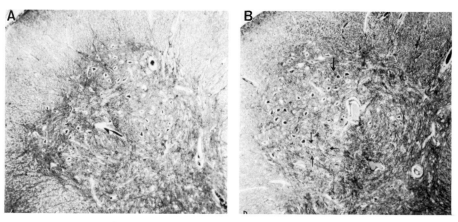

FIGURE 4.2   *Essentially normal anterior horns without inflammation in a section of a lumbar cord of a rapidly fatal human case of bulbar polio (A). In contrast, at another level of lumbar cord (B), foci of neuronophagia (arrows) and perivascular infiltrations are noted among many normal neurons. (Courtesy of Dr. A. Sabin.)*

Muscle and End-Plate Pathophysiology of Acute and Recovering Poliomyelitis

The acute destruction of the anterior horn cells leads to paralysis and subsequent atrophy of the muscles innervated by their respective motor neurons.

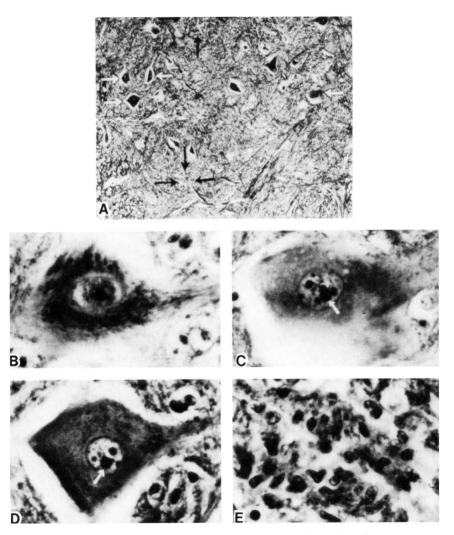

FIGURE 4.3 *Anterior horn in spinal cord of monkey sacrificed two days after spontaneous recovery from paralytic poliomyelitis of lower extremities; black arrows point to foci of glial neuronophagia, shown enlarged in (E) and white arrows point to neurons with diffuse chromatolysis and acidophilic intranuclear inclusions shown enlarged in (C) and (D) with arrows pointing to basophilic nucleoli. (B) One of only two almost normal neurons in (A). (Courtesy of Dr. A. Sabin.)*

The degree of paralysis and atrophy depends on the number of anterior horn cells that are either completely destroyed or partially affected. In the acute paralytic stage, the muscle fibers appear normal even though all of their motor neurons have been destroyed [24]. A few scattered inflammatory cells in the muscles have been seen but their presence does not correlate with the tenderness of muscles, a very common clinical finding [24]. The significance of this infiltrate in the acute disease is uncertain. Kakulas did not find such infiltrates, even when poliovirus was inoculated into the muscle [24].

The reduction in size of the paralyzed muscle fibers becomes evident within a few weeks after denervation. In the most severely wasted muscles, all of the motor units may be atrophic, but commonly, one or two isolated fascicles of 20–100 fibers may be of normal size, suggesting that their anterior horn cells escaped viral destruction [24]. All the paralyzed fibers become uniformly small if the denervation is complete. Often, however, the denervation is incomplete and there is variation of the muscle fiber size. The fibers with preserved innervation undergo hypertrophy and the number of fibers in the intact motor units increase and become tightly grouped due to collateral regeneration of distal nerve terminals. The small fibers in transverse sections are angulated and positive by the reduced nicotinamide adenine dinucleotide (NADH) dehydrogenase reaction. After four months of paralysis there is an increase in sarcolemmal nuclei, and by the sixth month, short linear rows of dark nuclei appear along with fat cells that are replacing degenerating fibers [24].

The damage of the anterior horn cells also results in secondary changes of the intramuscular nerves and the motor end-plates in both the acute and postacute disease. Chor found exactly the same changes in the motor nerve fiber and the motor end-plate of patients dying of poliomyelitis with the changes that occur in animals after a peripheral nerve section [25]. The only difference this author noted was that in poliomyelitis the changes were less uniform, possibly due to multisegmental innervation of skeletal muscle. Biopsies of the "motor points" studied by Woolf and Till in 1955 [26] showed degenerative changes in the collateral distal branches. They also found "hyperneurotized" fibers with extravagant plexuses and with as many as three end-plates that they attributed to abortive regenerative changes. They termed this phenomenon "chronic terminal motor neuropathy" and implied that the earliest changes were in the terminal portions of the surviving axons [26]. Further details of the anatomic changes in motor nerve endings in the muscles of patients with early poliomyelitis were reported by Carey et al. in 1944 using a metallic impregnation technique [27]. These authors found that the earliest morphologic change in the motor nerve fibers was a ball-like retraction of the terminal branches of the axis cylinders followed within 36 hours by granular degeneration and dissolution of many fibers of the end-plates. The degree of involvement was variable, being advanced in some fibers as early as twenty-six hours after the first symptoms or not perceptible in others. They suggested that in polio, degeneration of the nerve fiber proceeds centripetally, unlike the degeneration that follows a section of peripheral nerve where all the parts of the peripheral segment degenerate at the same time [27].

In the first several weeks of the disease, electromyography of the paralyzed muscle at rest is silent. Fibrillations develop in two to four weeks and persist indefinitely. The occurrence of fibrillation appears to correlate poorly with the degree of paresis [28–31], although the frequency of fibrillation seems to correlate with the extent of subsequent recovery [30]. At first the fibrillation potentials are of normal size, but as the muscle atrophies the fibrillation potentials become smaller in amplitude. Both fasciculations and even grouped fasciculations resembling myokymia can be detected [29,31].

Motor unit action potentials are reduced in numbers initially and an increase in polyphasia may be seen [29]. With improvement, the motor units become abnormally large in amplitude, with increased duration and polyphasia. The motor unit territory increases as was originally demonstrated by "synchrony" of motor units identified with two needles in the same muscle separated transversely by 2 centimeters or more [32,33]. This increase in size and territory is almost certainly due to sprouting of surviving motor units to reinnervate denervated muscle fibers; an additional mechanism of synchronization of motor units within the spinal cord has been suggested to explain synchrony in the acute stage [32,33]. Observations made late after acute disease have shown abnormalities of motor units even in muscles not initially suspected of weakness [6,17,34,35].

Conventional wisdom is that fibrillation is indicative of acute denervation. Although it is thought that in a simple nerve injury, fibrillation exists for months or at most a year or two, Buchthal and Pinelli showed that 20% of patients might have fibrillation five years after a nerve lesion [36]. Similarly, Lütschg and Ludin [37] showed fibrillation in three of twelve patients with nerve injuries six to sixteen years before. Fibrillation might be due to a continuing process of denervation and reinnervation as part of the "normal process" of repair after nerve injury. Wiechers has reported a case where fibrillations were continuously present nine years after polio [38]. Their presence in post-polio muscles does not appear to have any special implication because, as we have shown, they persist through the whole period, including the chronic state, in muscles that are strong, weak, stable, or deteriorating [6,9,17].

LONG-TERM CHANGES IN PATIENTS WITH POST-POLIO SYNDROME

Spinal Cord

Direct examination of the post-poliomyelitis spinal cord could provide insights into the status of motor neurons that have survived an acute viral insult and have been compensating for the lost neurons over a long period. This is of special neurobiologic interest, since changes in the spinal cord neurons are known only for the acute poliomyelitis and early convalescent periods [19–22,39] but not for a chronic postviral state. For this reason, we have reviewed, in a retrospective study, sections from the spinal cords from eight post-polio patients, ages thirty-six to sixty-one years, who died from non-neurological diseases nine months to forty-four years (mean 20.7 years) after the acute polio infection [9,15,16]. In an effort to understand the evolving changes of the surviving motor neurons in relation to the clinical symptomatology of the post-polio syndrome, we specifically sought to examine the spinal cords of both asymptomatic patients with stable post-polio deficits and no new symptoms (five patients), and patients who had PPMA that had started one to six years before death (three patients) [15,16]. An attempt was made to match the patients' clinical involvement in both groups with representative spinal cord sections. Concurrently examined control tissues were obtained from ten patients with ALS and five with spinocerebellar degeneration. Spinal cords from post-polio patients over the age of 61 years were excluded to avoid unspecific changes associated with aging [40]. All the material was selected from a large group of post-polio spinal cords taken from patients who, according to review of their charts, had a history of well-documented acute febrile paralytic illness in childhood or adolescence with partial recovery of motor function and subsequent stability. Seven patients had contracted polio during 1950 to 1952, and one in 1938. All the selected patients died from non-neuromuscular causes and had no associated neurological disease that could have potentially influenced the spinal cord morphology.

Six-micron transverse sections of paraffin-embedded spinal cords were selected from the cervical, thoracic, and lumbar regions to match the reported clinical condition of previously weakened and either stable or newly weakened muscles. Slides were coded and examined blindly without knowledge of the patients' clinical status (i.e., stable post-polio or PPMA) [9,15,16]. Sections were stained with hematoxylin and eosin and other routine histological stains, including Bodian's stain for axons and Cluver-Barrera and Woelcke stains for myelin. Particular attention was paid to pathologic signs of disease activity such as inflammation, gliosis, vascular, neuronal, and axonal changes. Inflammation and gliosis were graded as 1–4 based on their prominence. Thus, a few lymphocytes or reactive astrocytes were considered as grade 1, while brisk gliosis and/or marked inflammatory cell infiltrates were regarded as grade 4 changes [9,15,16].

Pathological changes were bilateral in six patients and included neuronal loss, atrophy of some motor neurons, active gliosis, and inflammation of variable degree (Figure 4.4). Complete destruction of the gray matter on one or both sides was noted at different levels in two patients, corresponding to a severe degree of residual paralysis. Motor neuron loss was present in all cases in the anteromedial and anterolateral groups of the gray matter. Several surviving neurons were present throughout the gray matter, but some of them had abnormal configuration of their somata consisting of atrophy, accumulation

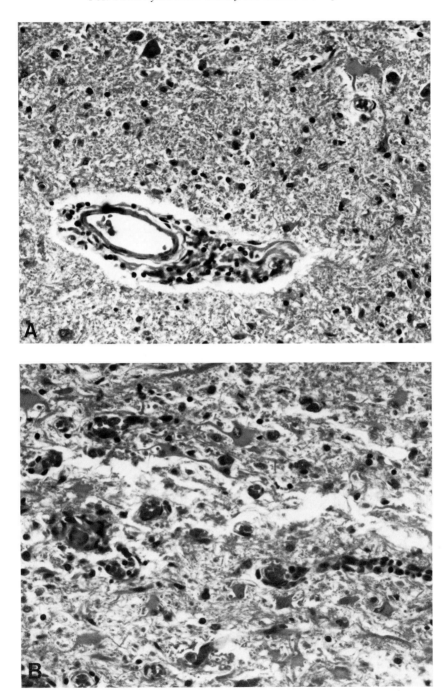

FIGURE 4.4 *Transverse sections of spinal cord from a patient who had acute polio forty-four years prior to death. Perivascular lymphocytic infiltrates (A) and gliosis (B) disproportional to the neuronal loss is noted (hematoxylin and eosin, × 100).*

of lipofuscin, and loss of Nissl substance. Inclusion bodies were not observed. Gliosis was most pronounced in one patient who died nine months after contracting polio, but some degree of reactive astrocytosis was present in all patients. The pathological findings in relation to the patients' clinical status are summarized in Table 4.5.

A remarkable finding was the presence of inflammation, which was perivascular in five and parenchymal in six of the spinal cords. The inflammatory exudates consisting of lymphocytes and plasma cells were present in every patient, regardless of the presence of new weakness (Table 4.5), suggesting that abnormalities continue for many years in the post-polio spinal cord (the site of the original viral infection). Prominent lymphocytic infiltration in the spinal cord has also been noted by Olsen and Plum in a patient one year after acute poliomyelitis [41]. Meningeal lymphocytic infiltration also was observed in almost all of our cases, decreasing in severity with time after the acute polio attack. In patients 6, 7, and 8, who had PPMA (Table 4.5), an additional finding was the presence of axonal spheroids (Figure 4.4B) (dystrophic axons) and occasional neurons with signs of chromatolysis. Axonal spheroids represent a defect in the movement of trophic material from the neuron down the body of the axon, and they are similar to the axonal swellings seen in b', b' iminodipropionitrile (IDPN) intoxication [42]. In motor neuron diseases they have been found predominantly in patients who have undergone recent (within six to twelve months) neuronal deterioration [43].

There was no evidence of corticospinal tract involvement, even when consecutive sections of each spinal cord segments were examined.

Our histopathological findings in PPMA differ from those found in ALS. In ALS, axonal spheroids are infrequent, gliosis is minimal, degeneration of the corticospinal tracts is always present, and inflammation is absent or rarely seen. Our findings suggest that many years after recovery and clinical stability, post-polio patients have signs of activity in their spinal cords that are unrelated to the presence of new muscle weakness [13]. The apparent ongoing neuronal activity complements our EMG findings that suggest a continuous remodeling of the motor unit until the ability of the surviving neurons for further sprouting ceases, resulting in new denervation and clinical muscle weakness as discussed below.

Muscle Biopsies

We have performed a total of 45 open muscle biopsies on 28 patients with new muscle weakness and six asymptomatic post-polio controls. Muscles at different stages of residual deficit were studied. These included newly symptomatic or asymptomatic muscles that had fully or partially recovered after the original illness or muscles originally spared, according to available clinical description, old photographs, or medical records. To our knowledge, none of the muscles examined by biopsy had been damaged by injury or needle insertions for at least six months before biopsy. Open muscle biopsy was performed according

Table 4.5   Summary of Clinicopathological Findings in the Spinal Cord of Post-Polio Patients

Patient	Age at Death (yr.)	Time After Acute Polio	Residual Deficit (No. of limbs)	Post-Polio Status	Pathological Findings[a]	
					Inflammation	Active Gliosis
1	36	3½ yr.	4	Stable	2+	3+
2	44	5½ yr.	4	Stable	2+	3+
3	44	9 mo.	4	Stable	4+	4+
4	46	23 yr.	2	Stable	2+	2+
5	59	29 yr.	2	Stable	2+	4
6	61	44 yr.	3	PPMA	4+	4[b]
7	58	31 yr.	2	PPMA	4+	4[b]
8	56	29 yr.	2	PPMA	2+	4[b]

[a]Grading of 1–4 according to the degree of abnormalities.
[b]Patients also had axonal spheroids and chromatolytic neurons (see text).

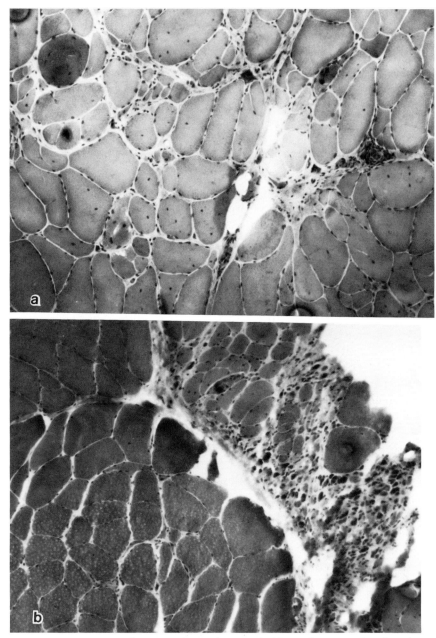

FIGURE 4.5   *Transverse frozen sections of a muscle biopsy from a patient in subgroup I stained with modified Gomori's trichrome. A mixture of myopathic (a) and neuropathic (b) features are noted. Increased connective tissue, variation of fiber size, hypertrophic fibers, several small round fibers, internal nuclei, and fiber splitting are often seen in (a). Old denervation with nuclear clumps and atrophic fibers in groups are noted in (b); occasional scattered angulated fibers are seen in the left fascicle (× 175).*

to standard techniques and specimens were fresh frozen in isopentane cooled to $-160°C$ with liquid nitrogen. Ten-micron sections of muscle were then processed for muscle enzyme histochemistry [47]. Serial muscle biopsy sections were also stained with trichrome, acid phosphatase, and esterase to characterize the type of inflammatory cells. During the follow-up study, post-polio patients who initially presented with new muscle weakness were re-examined by biopsy to assess changes in the muscles during progression of the disease [6–14].

The morphological features of each muscle are best described if subdivided into four different subgroups according to the condition of the sampled muscle:

Subgroup I: Muscles Originally Affected but Partially Recovered. Five biopsy samples were from muscles that were weak and atrophic from the original polio attack thirty to fifty years previously (mean patient age 48.5 years and mean interval after polio thirty-eight years) and recently had weakened further. The muscle in all patients showed a mixture of myopathic features along with new and old neurogenic changes (Figure 4.5), findings similar to those reported in chronic neurogenic conditions such as Charcot-Marie-Tooth disease, spinal muscular atrophy, and post-polio state [44–46]. Recent denervation is characterized by the presence of small scattered esterase-positive angulated fibers; chronic denervation is defined by the presence of fiber-type grouping of normal-sized fibers with or without atrophic fibers in groups [24–42]. The myopathic features consisted of increased connective tissue, occasional necrotic/phagocytosed fibers, variations of fiber size with big and small but rounded fibers, fiber splitting, and abundance of internal nuclei (Figure 4.5A). The neurogenic aspects were characterized by fiber type grouping, many nuclear clumps, groups of very small fibers (old group atrophy), and occasional small scattered angulated fibers (identical to those seen in Figure 4.6A) in the healthier areas of the muscle. The number of small scattered angulated fibers was variable, ranging from one to five per field of 100 fibers. A mild perivascular infiltration of inflammatory cells as well as interstitial inflammation (proportional to fiber necrosis and active phagocytosis) was noted in two of the biopsy samples.

Subgroup II: Muscles Originally Affected but Fully Recovered. These specimens, from patients with a mean age of 42.5 years (range thirty-three to fifty-six years), included biopsy samples from muscles that had fully regained the initially lost strength from poliomyelitis but recently had begun to lose it again. The predominant findings were signs of recent denervation with small, angulated fibers that tended to remain isolated and scattered among normal-sized fibers (Figure 4.6A) and the presence of extensive reinnervation with fiber-type grouping consisting of very large groups of up to 170 normal-sized fibers of each type (Figure 4.6B). The number of small scattered angulated fibers was quite variable, ranging from one to five per 100 fibers of normal size. Occasional nuclear clumps were noted and at times two to three adjacent atrophic fibers were seen (Figure 4.6A in this patient's follow-up biopsy). Mild perivascular inflammation was occasionally noted (as shown for subgroup III in Figure 4.7). Of interest is the muscle biopsy sample depicted in Figure 4.6C.

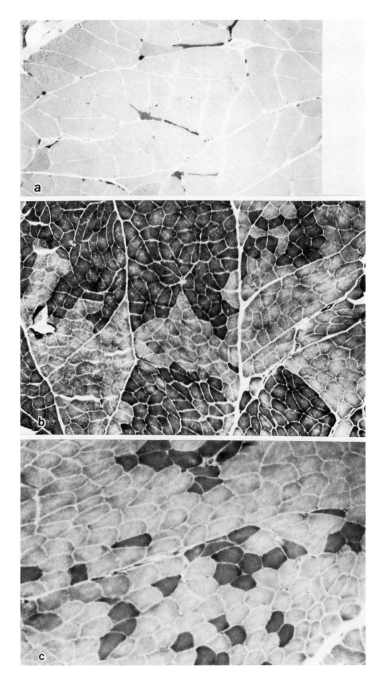

FIGURE 4.6 *Representative biopsy samples from subgroup II (see text). (a) Transverse frozen section of muscle biopsy stained with nonspecific esterase shows small scattered (dark) angulated fibers. Three atrophic fibers are adjacent, but group atrophy was absent (see text; ×175). (b) Biopsy sample from another patient, stained with NADH-TR, shows large fiber-type grouping of both fiber types (×85). (c) Grouping of type I (small groups) and type II (large groups) in a patient who eight years before this biopsy had only mild grouping and minimal symptoms. The new biopsy performed on the same muscle, which is now clinically weaker, reveals small groups of type I–composed fibers with few new angulated fibers noticeably absent eight years previously.*

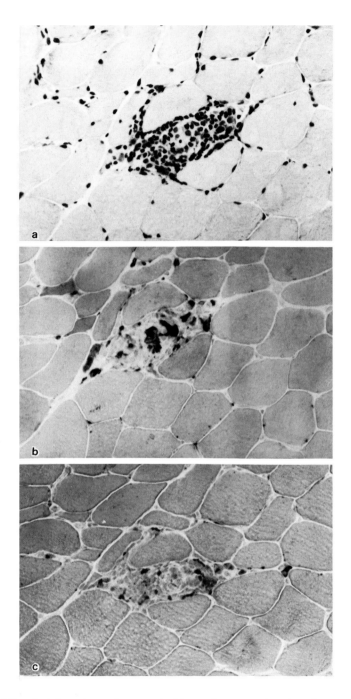

FIGURE 4.7 *Serial sections of a muscle biopsy from a patient in subgroup III stained with hematoxylin and eosin (a), esterase (b), and acid phosphatase (c). A perivascular lymphocytic infiltrate is noted that consists of very few esterase-positive cells (b), indicative of monocytes/activated T cells, and very rare acid phosphatase-positive cells (c), indicative of macrophages. Few scattered esterase-positive angulated fibers, indicative of recent de-nervation, are seen in (b) (×325; reproduced here at 75%).*

This muscle, examined by biopsy eight years previously, revealed mild grouping. The same muscle examined with a second biopsy eight years later because of new weakness, showed small groups of type I–composed fibers or predominance of large groups of type II–composed fibers along with few scattered angulated fibers (Figure 4.6C). One can hypothesize in this patient that the type I–fiber groups belong to weak neurons (as described below), with limited capacity to sprout and maintain large groups, resulting in early development of denervated (angulated) fibers when they reach their limit for further reinnervation. Their neighboring, apparently healthier neurons can maintain large groups but if they also reach their limit, they may not be able to rescue the denervated fibers of their neighboring weaker neurons and weakness ensues. Contrary to the previous subgroup I of examined muscles, clusters of atrophic fibers (old group atrophy) was rare even when the same muscle was re-examined by biopsy. This also contrasts to the findings in the weakening muscles of patients with ALS, in which the atrophic fibers always form groups (group atrophy), and the number of atrophic fibers in the groups increases rapidly until the whole fascicle atrophies, reflecting the death of whole neurons. Occasional atrophic fibers can lie adjacent to one another (Figure 4.6A), suggesting that as PPMA progresses, more such fibers may become atrophic, eventually producing a small group atrophy as more distal axonal sprouts that belong to the same or neighboring motor neurons continue to disintegrate. Development of such small group atrophy therefore represents either the end degeneration of a terminal and preterminal sprout that belonged to a large motor unit, or death of an entire small motor unit that emanated from a previously scarred neuron with limited capacity to reinnervate. Group atrophy was noted by Cashman et al. more frequently [34]. This we believe is most likely due to the selection of muscles examined by biopsy, since muscles that have been left weak or atrophic and have been symptomatic for many years are more likely to show group atrophy, as in subgroup I.

Subgroup III: Muscles Originally Spared Clinically but Newly Symptomatic.   These 16 patients had a mean age of 47.8 years (range thirty-four to sixty-eight). All had signs of residual weakness and atrophy in other extremities and had an illness that fulfilled the clinical criteria of PPMA. The predominant findings in these muscles were signs of chronic denervation/reinnervation with a large grouping (containing up to 150 normal-sized muscle fibers of each type), and the presence of occasional angulated small atrophic fibers scattered among normal-size fibers, in a pattern similar to that seen in subgroup II. The number of such angulated fibers was quite variable, ranging in general from one to three per 100 fibers of normal size. Contrary to the findings in subgroup II, however, hypertrophic fibers, internal nuclei, moth-eaten fibers, and fiber splitting were rare. Adjacent angulated atrophic fibers were not noted. Minimal interstitial or perivascular inflammation was noted in six of the sixteen biopsy samples (Figure 4.7).

Subgroup IV: Asymptomatic Post-Polio Patients.   Biopsies from five asymptomatic post-polio controls, mean age 44.1 years (range twenty-eight to fifty-four) included specimens from previously unaffected extremities (three patients) or from previously affected but subsequently recovered extremities (two patients). All five of these biopsy samples showed small to moderate-sized fiber-type grouping (up to fifty muscle fibers of each type), suggestive of a moderate degree of reinnervation but no signs of recent denervation, as evidenced by the absence of small angulated fibers. No inflammation was noted in this subgroup.

Immunohistochemical Findings on the Muscle Biopsy Specimens

Using specific antibodies to lymphocyte subsets we have recently found that muscle biopsies from PPMA patients have an increased number of lymphocytes as compared to other neurogenic diseases and ALS [48,49]. Some of these lymphocytes are CD4+ cells, but the majority are CD8+ cells surrounding muscle fibers that express major histocompatibility complex I-class antigen (MHC-I) on their surface. These findings suggest a possible T cell-mediated and MHC-I class restricted cytotoxic process.

One of the monoclonal antibodies we used, the anti-Leu-19, recognizes an N-CAM specific molecule that is expressed in the newly denervated muscle fibers but not in normal muscle. We found that in the muscle biopsy specimens from the PPMA patients there is a number of N-CAM-positive fibers that are of normal size; they are scattered and do not form groups. This indicates that the constant denervating process involves muscle fibers that have not yet become atrophic, but they are destined to be reinnervated if the collateral sprouts from the surviving motor neurons (that also have N-CAM) will make contact. Interestingly, the N-CAM-positive fibers in PPMA are mostly scattered and rarely in small groups, whereas in ALS they mostly form groups, suggesting that in PPMA there is denervation of single fibers due to deterioration of distal nerve terminals rather than denervation of groups of muscle fibers due to dropout of major axonal branches or whole neurons, as seen in ALS. These observations complement the single fiber electromyographic findings previously described [10].

PATHOGENESIS OF POST-POLIO SYNDROME

Immediately after recovery from acute polio, there exist unimpaired motor neurons, motor neurons that have fully recovered and can resume normal or near-normal function, motor neurons that have partially recovered (scarred neurons) with below normal ability to function, and dying neurons (Figure 4.8). The terminal axons of the surviving motor neurons begin to sprout in an attempt to reinnervate the muscle fibers orphaned by the death of their parent neurons (Figure 4.9). During this process, an uninvolved or recovered anterior horn cell adopts in its motor unit territory additional muscle fibers that could potentially extend up to four to five new muscle fibers for every muscle fiber

1. Normal (non-stressed)

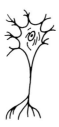

2. Normal, previously unaffected, but now stressed

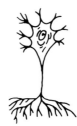

3. "Normal"-looking, fully recovered but smaller in size; overstressed

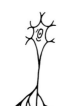

4. "Scarred", incompletely recovered, overstressed

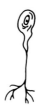

FIGURE 4.8   *Status of remaining neurons after recovery from acute paralytic poliomyelitis.*

originally innervated [50]. This indicates that theoretically a single motor neuron originally innervating an average of 200 fibers may eventually become responsible for innervating 800–1000 fibers. This potentially taxing process produces large motor units and is so effective that despite the loss of up to 50% of the original number of motor neurons the muscle can retain clinically normal strength as we previously discussed [9].

However, the ability of the remaining neurons to oversprout and recruit additional muscle fibers in their territory and maintain the metabolic needs of all their distal nerve terminals on a long-term basis depends on the integrity and functional capacity of each neuronal soma in an affected spinal cord segment. On this basis, the post-polio spinal cord can be considered theoretically as containing four subsets of neurons, as illustrated in Figure 4.8: (1) the normal, nonstressed neurons present in a spinal cord territory with minimal original disease—such neurons do not need to compensate for lost or possibly dysfunctioning surrounding neurons; (2) the normal previously unaffected neurons present in a territory of affected neurons—these cells compensate for the lost ones and are being stressed to oversprout and recruit denervated muscle fibers in their territory; (3) the previously affected but seemingly completely recovered neurons that are smaller than normal and have below normal capacity

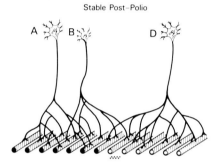

FIGURE 4.9 *Representation of remaining neurons after acute polio and in the chronic post-polio state. In the stable post-polio, there is continuing remodeling of the motor unit by effective reinnervation of the newly denervated fibers. In early PPMA there are only small scattered angulated fibers (dark) representing disintegration of distal sprouts corresponding to early new muscle weakness. As PPMA progresses, contiguous muscle fibers can become denervated and hence possible development of atrophic fibers in small groups (dark fibers), which represent the end stage of PPMA in that muscle. Dots represent the nuclear clumps that remained since the acute polio attack.*

for axonal sprouting; and (4) the scarred, incompletely recovered neurons that control a few muscle fibers and have marginal ability to maintain new axonal terminals.

After maximum recovery is achieved following acute polio, the reinnervated motor units are not matured and stabilized as expected. To the contrary, as suggested by the presence of abnormal jitter and blocking in all the muscles regardless of the presence of new weakness [9,17,34], there is an ongoing denervating/reinnervating process resulting in a continuous remodeling of the motor units (Figure 4.9), even in muscles with stable muscle strength because at a given time there are more denervated fibers that possibly could be reinnervated. This process, which reflects a continuing attempt of the post-polio motor neuron to reinnervate additional muscle fibers via excessive distal sprouting, has been stressing the cell body for a number of years. When the capabilities of the motor neuron to maintain this excess of functional sprouts reach a limit, the neurons can no longer maintain the metabolic demand of all their sprouts and lose their ability to reinnervate further. As a result, slow deterioration affects the nerve terminals. This process, which in essence reflects neuronal metabolic endurance, takes place in all the neurons but it is more taxing first to the scarred and smaller neurons and proceeds slowly to the healthiest neurons as illustrated in Figures 4.8 and 4.9. As more sprouts degenerate and the orphaned newly denervated muscle fibers cannot be recruited by the neighboring neurons with already saturated motor units, permanent denervation ensues (dark fibers in Figure 4.9).

The collateral sprouting mechanism experimentally demonstrated by Pestronk [51,52] involves the ultraterminal sprouts that originate from a distal nerve terminal arborization to reinnervate the neighboring denervated muscle fibers and the preterminal sprouts that originate from the intact axon beyond the original end plate (Figure 4.10). Based on the histological and immunohistochemical findings discussed above and our previously reported electrophysiological findings of jitter, neurogenic jitter, and blocking [6,9,17], it appears that in PPMA the ultraterminal sprouts most likely disintegrate first, followed by the preterminal sprouts. This is based on our finding that neurogenic jitter, which is present in ALS but absent in PPMA, originates more proximally, at the axonal branch points. As each terminal dies and muscle fibers are no longer reinnervated, weakness appears that progresses slowly.

As an example of this, one can imagine a situation discussed previously [9] where there are 801 fibers coupled to one neuron intrinsically capable of innervating only 800 fibers. Subsequently, that fiber will be innervated by a new sprout that could form an effective synapse and an old sprout will die. There will always be one fiber not innervated. As the neuron loses its ability to keep pace, a muscle fiber will lose its innervation and not be reinnervated. Taken en masse, it is only at this time that muscles as a whole lose their strength. This scenario summarized in Figure 4.10(1) is consistent with (1) increased jitter and blocking even in asymptomatic patients, which does not correlate with disease activity but reflects the continuing denervating/

FAILURE OF COLLATERAL SPROUTING IN PARTIAL DENERVATION

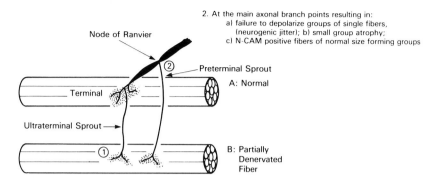

FIGURE 4.10   *Examples of collateral sprouting in a normal* (A) *and partially denervated fiber* (B) *via terminal, preterminal, and ultraterminal sprouts as could occur in PPMA. (1) and (2) correspond to potential areas of dysfunction within the motor unit, along with the expected histological, immunocytochemical and electrophysiological feature. The findings favor a distal axonal degeneration (1) rather than a more proximal process within the motor unit (2), as discussed in the text.*

reinnervating process; (2) the presence of new scattered angulated fibers in the muscle biopsy sample, which is a sign of recent denervation and coincides with the presence of new symptoms; (3) the presence of scattered N-CAM-positive fibers of normal size; (4) fall of macro-EMG amplitude, which drops as weakness progresses, indicative of muscle fiber loss in the motor unit [53]; and (5) the absence of neurogenic jitter. Neurogenic jitter, characterized by groups of action potentials that jitter together, is ascribed to axonal branch points, and it can be observed in ALS [17]. Its absence in our patients with PPMA supports the observation that axonal twigs rather than the whole nerve are first affected, as depicted in Figure 4.9(2). Furthermore, if major axonal branches or entire neurons were dying as in ALS, atrophic fibers in groups (group atrophy) and groups of N-CAM-positive fibers would have developed, resulting in more severe and rapidly progressive muscle weakness.

As PPMA progresses, however, some adjacent fibers will become atrophic (as noted in Figure 4.6 in a follow-up muscle biopsy sample from a PPMA patient) and eventually small group atrophy will develop as more distal preterminal and ultraterminal sprouts that belong to the same or neighboring motor units disintegrate (Figures 4.8 and 4.9). Finally, some of the scarred neurons with minimal muscle reserves, such as those innervating few muscle fibers, may completely disintegrate, resulting in new group atrophy. Group atrophy therefore represents the end stage of this process and, as noted by others [34], it can be seen in post-polio muscle biopsy samples. This process is depicted in Figure 4.9, summarizing our clinico-histological profile of the post-polio state, including early and late signs of disintegration of the distal nerve terminals. Based on the electrophysiological instability of clinically stable post-polio muscles and the histological signs of inflammation, neuronal chromatolysis, and relative smallness of many surviving neurons even in the stable post-polio state, it seems that PPMA represents the tip of the iceberg in continuously dysfunctioning neurons, clinically manifested when neuronal reserves have diminished, more nerve terminals cannot survive, and further reinnervation cannot take place.

Normal aging alone cannot be the cause of PPMA because neuronal loss does not occur in people under sixty years of age [40] and muscle biopsy specimens from normal people who are under seventy years of age rarely show small angulated fibers [54]. In addition, all the patients we selected to study were under sixty years of age (average forty-seven years) in order to avoid the effect of aging. Epidemiological data also indicate that it is the length of the interval between onset of acute polio and the appearance of new symptoms that is a determining variable for PPMA, not the chronological age [55]. PPMA appears to express itself clinically approximately thirty years after the original polio attack, which suggests that the remaining overstressed post-polio neurons may succumb earlier to the normal aging process or may even have a shorter life span. Motor unit decompensation may be accelerated by normal aging, which has been associated with increased end-plate complexity and reduced terminal sprouting [52,56]. Therefore, premature aging brought on by attrition could be the main cause explaining the mechanisms discussed above. This is the theory we favor at the moment.

The possibility that immune or viral mechanisms may also play a role in the pathogenesis of PPMA, although unlikely, cannot be excluded. We have found a few such indications but their significance is uncertain.

1. A mild inflammatory response occurs in up to 40% of the PPMA muscles examined. Inflammation, mostly lymphocytes, was in areas unrelated to muscle fiber necrosis or phagocytosis, at times was perivascular, and at other times resembled a lymphorrhage, similar to those rarely observed in myasthenia gravis, a disease of immunopathologic origin. In addition, many of the muscle fibers express MHC-I class antigen on their surface, suggestive of T cell-mediated and MHC-I restricted cytotoxic process. Three of our PPMA patients who had significant inflammatory response in the muscle biopsy samples resembling inflammatory myopathy were treated with corticosteroids or interferon but with no response [1–14,57].

2. Weak oligoclonal IgG bands of unknown origin were noted in the CSF of some PPMA patients.

3. There were signs of an active process in the spinal cords of post-polio patients up to forty-four years after the original polio attack. These included inflammation, gliosis, neuronal chromatolysis, and axonal spheroids. Although

polio virus is a cytolytic RNA virus, and poliomyelitis is a monophasic disease with no activity in the spinal cord neurons beyond the first six months, poliovirus can cause a persistent infection in animals or immunosuppressed humans [58,59]. It is possible, therefore, that after the viral attack on the motor neurons took its original toll on a number of neurons, some residual "sparks" could have caused an indolent but continuous inflammation in the surviving neurons, leading to a subclinical neuronal dysfunction. Whether these sparks represent residual viral genomes and whether PPMA is a slow viral illness remains to be determined using in situ hybridization and polymerase chain reaction. Alternatively, the inflammation in the muscle and spinal cord could have been simply a nonspecific response to a continuous mechanical overstress of the weak limbs or a nonspecific reaction of neurons to their disintegrating distal axonal sprouts.

REFERENCES

1. Dalakas MC, Sever JL, Madden DL, et al. Late post-poliomyelitis muscular atrophy: clinical, virological, and immunological studies. Rev Infect Dis 1984;6:S562.
2. Dalakas MC, Sever JL, Fletcher M, et al. Neuromuscular symptoms in patients with old poliomyelitis: clinical, virological and immunological studies. In: Halstead LS, Wiechers DO, eds. Late effects of poliomyelitis. Miami: Symposia Foundation, 1984, p 73.
3. Dalakas MC. Post-poliomyelitis muscular atrophy. In: Laurie G, Raymond J, eds. Proceedings of the 2nd international poliomyelitis and independent living conference. St. Louis: CV Mosby, 1984, p 18.
4. Dalakas MC. Recent research issues in post-poliomyelitis muscular atrophy (PPMA): pathogenesis and rate of progression. In: Laurie G, Raymond J, eds. Proceedings of third international post-polio conference. St. Louis: Gazette International Networking Institute, 1986, p 39.
5. Dalakas MC. New neuromuscular symptoms in patients with old poliomyelitis: a three year follow-up study. Eur Neurol 1986;25:381.
6. Dalakas MC, Elder G, Hallet M, et al: A long-term follow-up study of patients with post-poliomyelitis neuromuscular symptoms. N Engl J Med 1986;314:959.
7. Dalakas MC. New neuromuscular symptoms after polio (the post-polio syndrome): clinical studies and pathologic mechanisms. In: Halstead LS, Wiechers DO, eds. Research and clinical aspects of the late effects of poliomyelitis, Vol 23. White Plains, NY: March of Dimes, 1987, p 241.
8. Dalakas MC. Post-polio syndrome. In: Yearbook of nursing '88. Springhouse, PA: Springhouse, 1988, pp 50–4.
9. Dalakas MC, Hallett M. The post-polio syndrome. In: Plum F, ed. Advances in contemporary neurology. Philadelphia: FA Davis, 1988, pp 51–94.
10. Dalakas MC, Elder G, Cunningham G, et al. Morphological changes in the muscles of patients with post-poliomyelitis muscular atrophy (PPMA): analysis of 38 biopsies. Neurology 1986;36:137.
11. Dalakas MC, Elder G, Hallett M, et al. Post-poliomyelitis neuromuscular symptoms. N Engl J Med 1986;315:897.
12. Dalakas MC. Morphological changes in the muscles of patients with post-poliomyelitis new weakness. A histochemical study of 39 muscle biopsies. Presented at the VI international congress on neuromuscular diseases, Los Angeles, July 1986. Muscle Nerve 1986;9:117.

13. Dalakas MC. ALS and post-polio: differences and similarities. In: Halstead LS, Wiechers DO, eds. Research and clinical aspects of the late effects of poliomyelitis, Vol 23. White Plains, NY: March of Dimes, 1987, p 63.

14. Dalakas MC. Morphological changes in the muscles of patients with post-poliomyelitis neuromuscular symptoms. Neurology 1988;38:99–104.

15. Pezeshkpour GH, Dalakas MC. Pathology of spinal cord in post-poliomyelitis muscle atrophy. In: Halstead LS, Wiechers DO, eds. Research and clinical aspects of the late effects of poliomyelitis, Vol 23. White Plains, NY: March of Dimes, 1987, pp 229–36.

16. Pezeshkpour GH, Dalakas MC. Long-term changes in the spinal cord of patients with old poliomyelitis: signs of continuous disease activity. Arch Neurol 1988;45:505–8.

17. Ravits J, Hallett M, Baker M, et al. Clinical and electromyographic studies of post-poliomyelitis muscular atrophy. Neurology 1987;37:161.

18. Dalakas MC. Post-poliomyelitis motor neuron disease: What did we learn in reference to amyotrophic lateral sclerosis? In: Hudson A, ed. Amyotrophic lateral sclerosis. Toronto: Toronto University Press, 1990, pp. 326–57.

19. Bodian D. Histopathologic basis of clinical findings in poliomyelitis. Am J Med 1949;6:563.

20. Bodian D. Poliomyelitis: pathological anatomy. In: Poliomyelitis: papers and discussions presented at the first international poliomyelitis conference. Philadelphia: JB Lippincott, 1949, p 62.

21. Bodian D. Poliomyelitis. In: Minckler J, ed. Pathology of the nervous system, Vol 3. New York: McGraw-Hill, 1982, p 2323.

22. Bodian D. Motorneuron disease and recovery in experimental poliomyelitis. In: Halstead LS, Wiechers DO, eds. Late effects of poliomyelitis. Miami: Symposia Foundation, 1984, p 45.

23. Price RW, Plum F. Poliomyelitis. In: Vinken PJ, Bruyn GW, eds. Handbook of clinical neurology, Vol 34. New York: Elsevier, 1978, p 93.

24. Kakulas BA, Adams RD. Diseases of muscle. Philadelphia: Harper & Row, 1985, p 734–9.

25. Chor H. Nerve degeneration in poliomyelitis: changes in the motor nerve endings. Arch Neurol Psychiatry 1933; 29:344–58.

26. Woolf AL, Till K. The pathology of the lower motor neuron in the light of the new muscle biopsy techniques. Proc R Soc Med 1953;48:189–98.

27. Carey EJ, Massopust LC, Zeit W, et al. Anatomic changes in motor nerve endings in human muscle in early poliomyelitis. J Neuropathol Exp Neurol 1944;3:121–30.

28. Daube JR. Electrophysiologic studies in the diagnosis and prognosis of motor neuron diseases. Neurol Clin 1985;3:473.

29. Goodgold J, Eberstein A. Electrodiagnosis of neuromuscular diseases. Baltimore: Williams & Wilkins, 1972.

30. Hertz H, Madsen A, Buchthal F. Prognostic implications of electromyography in acute anterior poliomyelitis. J Bone Joint Surg 1954;36A:902.

31. Kimura J. Electrodiagnosis in diseases of nerve and muscle. Philadelphia: FA Davis, 1983.

32. Buchthal F, Clemmesen S. On the differentiation of muscle atrophy by electromyography. Acta Psychiatr Neurol 1941;16:143.

33. Buchthal F, Honke P. Electromyographic examination of patients suffering from poliomyelitis. Acta Med Scand 1944;116:148.

34. Cashman NR, Maselli R, Wollman RL, et al. Late denervation in patients with antecedent paralytic poliomyelitis. N Engl J Med 1987;317:7.

35. Cruz Martinez A, Perez Conde MC, Ferrer MT. Chronic partial denervation is

more widespread than is suspected clinically in paralytic poliomyelitis: electrophysiological study. Eur Neurol 1983;22:314.

36. Buchthal F, Pinelli P. Action potentials in muscular atrophy of neurogenic origin. Neurology [Minneapolis] 1953;3:591.
37. Lütschg J, Ludin HP. Electromyographic findings in patients after recovery from peripheral nerve lesions and poliomyelitis. J Neurol 1981;225:25.
38. Wiechers DO. New concepts of the reinnervated motor unit. Muscle Nerve 1987;10:661.
39. Peers JH. The pathology of convalescent poliomyelitis. Am J Pathol 1943;19:673.
40. Tomlinson BE, Irving D. The numbers of limb motor neurons in the human lumbosacral cord throughout life. J Neurol Sci 1977;34:213.
41. Plum F, Olsen ME. Myelitis and myelopathy. In: Baker AB, Baker LH, eds. Clinical neurology, Vol 3. Hagerstown, Md.: Harper & Row, 1973, p 1.
42. Griffin JW, Price DL. Proximal axonopathies induced by toxic chemicals. In: Spencer PS, Schaumburg HH, eds. Experimental and clinical neurotoxicology. Baltimore: Williams & Wilkins, 1980, p 161.
43. Carpenter S. Proximal axonal enlargement in motor neuron disease. Neurology 1968;18:842.
44. Drachman DB, Murphy SR, Nigam MP, et al. Myopathic changes in chronically denervated muscle. Arch Neurol 1967;16:14–24.
45. Haase GR, Shy GM. Pathological changes in muscle biopsies from patients with peroneal muscular atrophy. Brain 1960;83:631.
46. Lucas GJ, Forester FM. Charcot-Marie-Tooth disease with associated myopathies: a report of a family. Neurology 1962;12:629–38.
47. Engel WK. Selective and nonselective susceptibility of muscle fiber types: a new approach to human neuromuscular diseases. Arch Neurol 1979;22:97–117.
48. Dalakas M, Illa I. The post-polio syndrome. In: Rowland LP, ed. Motor neuron diseases. New York: Raven Press, 1990 (in press).
49. Illa I, Dalakas M. Immunocytochemical changes in the muscle of patients with postpoliomyelitis muscular atrophy (PPMA): relevance to amyotrophic lateral sclerosis (ALS) (abstract). Neurology 1990;40(S)428.
50. Sharrad WJW. Correlation between changes in the spinal cord and muscle paralysis in poliomyelitis. Proc R Soc Med 1953;40:346.
51. Pestronk A, Drachman DB. Sprouting and regeneration of motor nerves. In: Schotland DL, ed. Disorders of the motor unit. New York: Wiley, 1982, p 173.
52. Pestronk A, Drachman DB, Griffin JW. Effects of aging on nerve sprouting and regeneration. Exp Neurol 1980;70:65.
53. Maselli RA, Cashman N, Salazar E, et al. Impairment of neuromuscular transmission in patients with prior history of poliomyelitis. Muscle Nerve 1987;10:665.
54. Hicks JE, Cutler NA, Dalakas MC. Assessment of peripheral nervous system involvement in normal aged and Alzheimer's patients (abstract). Arch Phys Med Rehabil 1985;16:10.
55. Halstead LS, Wiechers DO, eds. Research and clinical aspects of the late effects of poliomyelitis, Vol 23. White Plains, NY: March of Dimes, 1987.
56. Rosenheimer JL, Smith DO. Differential changes in the end-plate architecture of functionally diverse muscle during aging. J Neurophysiol 1985;53:1567.
57. Dalakas MC, Aksamit AJ, Madden DL, et al. Recombinant a_2 interferon in a pilot trial of patients with ALS. Arch Neurol 1986;43:933.
58. Davis LF, Bodian D, Price DL, et al. Chronic progressive poliomyelitis secondary to vaccination of an immunodeficient child. N Engl J Med 1977;297:241.
59. Miller JR. Prolonged intracerebral infection with poliovirus in asymptomatic mice. Ann Neurol 1981;9:590.

Chapter 5

The Electrophysiologic Characteristics of the Late Progressive Polio Syndrome

John J. Kelly, Jr.

The syndrome of late progression of neuromuscular symptoms in patients with otherwise stable polio is one of the major public health problems in this country. Patients who are otherwise productive and have recovered from polio in early childhood or young adulthood gradually become weak and dysfunctional with varying amounts of pain and fatigue [1–7]. On the face of it, clarification of this disorder should be a relatively simple task because the etiology, target organ, and sequelae of polio are well known. Yet, this syndrome has defied our understanding. In this chapter, we will review the physiology of acute and recovered polio and review what is known of the late effects of polio as seen by the electrophysiologist.

PHYSIOLOGY

Acute poliomyelitis causes widespread anterior horn cell death [8]. Clinical, electrophysiologic, and pathologic studies show that damage affects segments of the spinal cord in a multifocal fashion [9]. For example, all of the L3, L4 muscles of the hip girdle may be affected in one leg, whereas the L5 through S2 muscles are affected in the other leg. Although seemingly localized to clinically affected segments of the spinal cord, anterior horn cell loss is more widespread and subclinical loss is present in other limbs not known to have been originally involved. This is evident in virtually all old-polio patients studied by subsequent EMG of unaffected muscles.

Acute anterior horn cell death results in denervation of all of the scattered muscle fibers belonging to an individual motor unit (Figure 5.1). If only a few anterior horn cells supplying a muscle die, weakness is transient or not noticed by the patient and reinnervation rapidly occurs by preterminal sprouting of

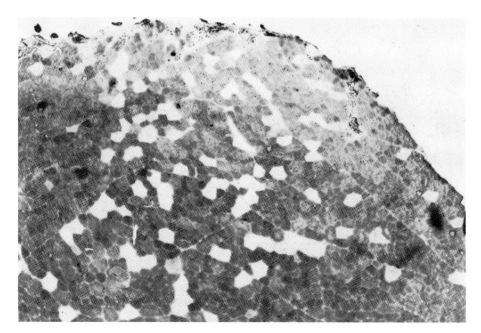

FIGURE 5.1   *A cross-section of muscle showing the distribution of PAS-negative muscle fibers, which belong to a single motor unit, as demonstrated by the glycogen-depletion technique (×40; reproduced here at 75%). (Reprinted with permission from Edstrom and Kugelberg [10].)*

adjacent motor unit axons (Figure 5.2). The denervated muscle fibers are quickly incorporated into the healthy surviving motor units. Although patients with mild polio may recall a febrile illness during the peak polio periods, they may not recall weakness of an extremity. However, subsequent careful EMG examination will reveal evidence of loss of even a few motor units with characteristic enlargement of surviving motor units due to reinnervation [11,12].

More severe loss of anterior horn cells results in partial or complete denervation of muscles in a segmental (myotomal) distribution. Surviving anterior horn cells, however, have a remarkable capacity for sprouting and reinnervating denervated muscle fibers. It has been estimated that 50% or more of the anterior horn cells can be lost, yet the remainder of the anterior horn cells can still achieve complete reinnervation of muscle fibers with resulting normal strength [13]. Subsequent EMG will reveal marked enlargement of motor unit potentials in this setting—the so-called giant motor unit potentials of old polio [14].

Muscles innervated by segments of spinal cord with more severe or total loss of anterior horn cells recover incompletely or not at all. Here, fibrillation potentials (Figure 5.3), representing spontaneous depolarizations of denervated muscle fibers, will persist in addition to giant motor unit potentials of reinnervation. Eventually, most of the denervated muscle fibers degenerate and atro-

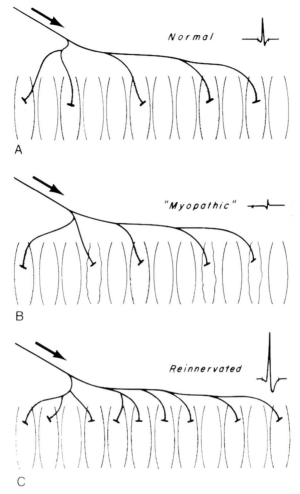

FIGURE 5.2 *Schematic depiction of motor unit anatomy and corresponding motor unit potential in normal (A), myopathic (B), and reinnervated (C) muscle. (Reprinted with permission from Adams and Victor [9].)*

phy with muscle fibrosis. Chronic, weakened muscles typically have areas of fibrosis alternating with areas of giant motor unit potentials. Occasionally, small atrophic muscle fibers can survive indefinitely with fibrillation potentials that are very small due to atrophy of the muscle fibers generating the potentials.

MOTOR UNIT CHARACTERISTICS

Accurate data on the physiology of motor units in reinnervated and normal human muscle are important to understanding recovery from polio. Although

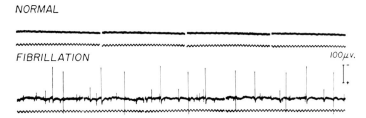

FIGURE 5.3   *Normally, with the EMG electrode resting quietly in muscle, there is no spontaneous activity. With denervation (bottom), fibrillation potentials appear, representing the spontaneous discharges of individual denervated muscle fibers. (Reprinted by permission of Mayo Foundation [14].)*

human data are sparse, it is possible to combine animal data on motor unit characteristics with electrophysiologic studies of human muscle to arrive at a "best guess" as to likely characteristics of normal muscle and changes in motor units that occur with reinnervation.

Early electrophysiologic work on motor unit characteristics was done by Erminio et al. [15,16], who used concentric multielectrode needles to study motor units in normal human limb muscles. They found that the motor units in limb muscles varied from 5 to 10 millimeters in mean diameter (Figure 5.4). Patients with denervating-reinnervating diseases had increased voltage over active electrode sites, suggesting increased fiber density at the sites. Yet, there was a relatively small increase in motor unit diameter, which was greatest (up to 140%) in patients with the chronic degenerative disease of the anterior horn cells (amyotrophic lateral sclerosis). They felt that this increase in motor unit territory was not due to sprouting but was more likely due to the synchronous firing of two or more motor units.

Edstrom and Kugelberg [9] then studied individual motor unit anatomy in normal animals using the glycogen depletion technique (Figure 5.1). They stimulated individual nerve fibers supplying single motor units at very high rates for long periods. Muscle fibers belonging to the stimulated motor unit were selectively depleted of their glycogen content and subsequent histochemical staining disclosed the distribution of the glycogen-depleted muscle fibers belonging to the motor unit. They found that the territory of normal motor units averaged 12% to 26% of the cross-sectional area of a muscle with highest density in the center of the motor unit and a gradual drop-off to the periphery [18]. In denervated-reinnervated muscles, they found that reinnervated motor units had the same or even a slightly decreased cross-sectional area with an increased fiber density and preservation of the same central concentration of muscle fibers. Thus, despite the fact that there had been considerable sprouting, as judged by progressively larger groups of adjacent muscle fibers of the same histochemical type, there was little evidence for extensive enlargement of the

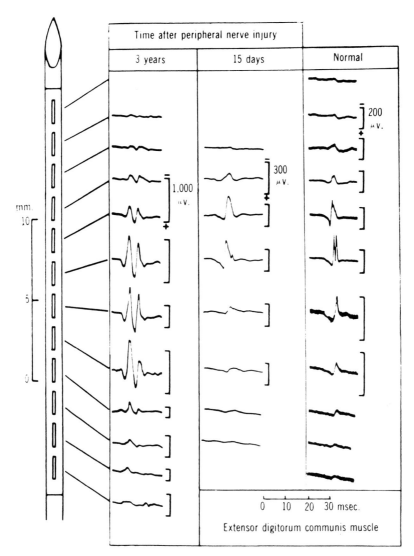

FIGURE 5.4   *Schematic diagram of a multielectrode and corresponding motor unit activity in muscle at different intervals after peripheral nerve injury. Despite an increase in voltage at active sites due to reinnervation and increased fiber density, the diameter of the motor unit changes minimally over time. (Reprinted with permission from Erminio et al. [15].)*

cross-sectional area and no evidence for subunit formation. They suggested that Erminio and colleagues' [15] findings of enlarged motor units in ALS patients may have been due to technical factors.

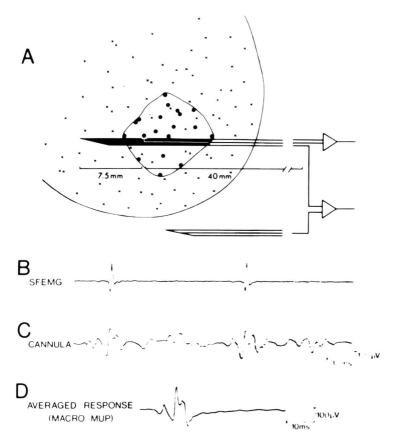

FIGURE 5.5   *Schematic depiction (A) of SF-EMG electrode and macro-EMG electrode in a motor unit. The macro-EMG electrode spans almost the entire motor unit. The SF-EMG potential (B) is correspondingly small and simple, whereas the macro-EMG potential (D) is larger and more complex, representing the summated activity from the whole motor unit. (C) Recording from the cannula. (Reprinted with permission from Stalberg and Trontelj [17].)*

EMG Techniques

Further clarification of normal and abnormal motor unit anatomy occurred with the introduction of single-fiber (SF) EMG techniques as applied by Stalberg and Trontelj [17]. As opposed to concentric electrodes, which can only record from several fibers of a motor unit and are unable to isolate individual muscle fiber potentials, single fiber techniques have the advantage of more selective recordings than concentric needle electrodes and can record individual muscle fiber potentials, thereby providing accurate information regarding the distribution of muscle fibers within an individual motor unit (Figure 5.5). This technique, by making accurate counts of fiber density and distribution of muscle fibers within a motor unit possible for the first time in humans, disclosed a maximal motor unit diameter of 6 millimeters in the forearm finger extensor

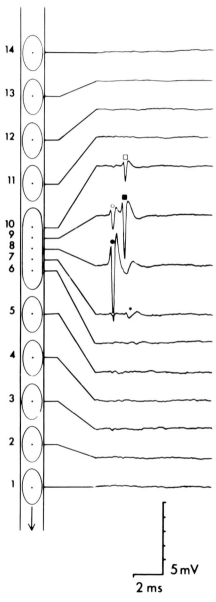

5 mV

2 ms

FIGURE 5.6 *Schematic depiction of SF-multielectrode and the corresponding activity recorded at each electrode position from a normal muscle. This allows estimates of fiber density at each site, the distribution of fibers within a motor unit, and the cross-sectional size of motor units. (Reprinted with permission from Stalberg [19].)*

muscle [20] (Figure 5.6), a value that agrees with data from Erminio et al. [15]. In agreement with Edstrom and Kugelberg, Schwartz et al. [21] found a markedly increased fiber density in the reinnervated muscle in ALS patients, but no increase in motor unit territory or motor unit area. Later, morphologic work by Slack and Pockett [22] using denervated intercostal rat muscle disclosed that sprouting is "a local response to a local stimulus." In their study, sprouts traveled only about 100 microns from a nerve terminal to innervate denervated muscle fibers and few if any sprouts traveled beyond 200 microns.

EMG Results

Based on this work, we can now make an educated guess as to motor unit characteristics in normal and reinnervated limb muscles. Normal motor units in limb muscles probably vary from about 5 to 10 millimeters in diameter. There is a higher fiber density in the center of motor units in normal muscle

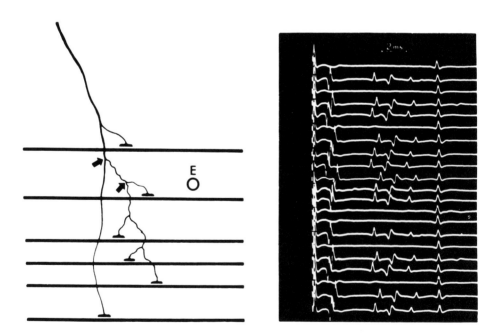

FIGURE 5.7   *Schematic depiction of the reinnervation of newly denervated muscle by axonal sprouting (arrows). These sprouts are initially small and immature, and conduct slowly and somewhat uncertainly. As a result, the SFEMG potentials recorded (right) are complex with late components. In addition, when conduction fails at the site of the arrows, the entire subsequent train of late components drops out. This is called* neurogenic blocking *to distinguish it from the blocking that occurs in neuromuscular transmission disorders. (Reprinted with permission from Stalberg and Trontelj [17].)*

with a gradual drop-off in fiber density from the center to the periphery. Reinnervated motor units in motor neuron diseases are likely the same size cross-sectionally as normal motor units. However, fiber density is markedly increased. Sprouting is thus a local phenomenon and sprouts probably do not reach distances of greater than two to three muscle fiber diameters (100–150 microns) from the originating nerve terminal. As a result, successful reinnervation due to sprouting results in survival of muscle fibers within the immediate vicinity of innervated muscle fibers. This probably accounts for the large groups of atrophic, denervated muscle fibers sometimes bounded by fascicular margins that are seen in old-polio patients next to other areas where reinnervation apparently has been complete. Sprouts from adjacent intact units cannot enter and reinnervate these large, atrophic fiber bundles, nor can they cross fascicular boundaries.

Single-fiber EMG studies and clinical experience suggest that early neuromuscular connections due to sprouting are immature and unstable [17]. Initially, these newly incorporated single-muscle fiber potentials are widely separated from the main bulk of the motor unit potential (Figure 5.7) not due to distance but due to slow conduction in axon sprouts that are thin and poorly myelinated. In addition, these sprouts are unable to transmit rapid trains of impulses due to their increased refractory period. Also, release of acetylcholine is defective at immature nerve terminals, and neuromuscular transmission fails. The motor unit potential has widely dispersed components that are unstable (jitter), and that frequently fail to fire (block). This causes fatigue and weakness. As the motor unit matures, these sprouts enlarge, the myelin coating thickens, and impulse and neuromuscular transmission improves. Gradually, these late components become more stable and are incorporated into the bulk of the motor unit. Blocking, when it occurs, tends to be neurogenic in nature (Figure 5.7). With time (greater than six months), further incorporation of these components into the body of the main motor unit occurs and blocking ceases. Eventually (over a year or more), the typical giant potentials of old polio appear. Patients then enter the stable phase of either partially or completely recovered polio.

REINNERVATION FACTORS

Although reinnervation due to preterminal sprouting, as occurs in polio or other anterior horn cell (AHC) diseases, is now better understood, many questions remain. What is the stimulus that provokes sprouting? Why is sprouting limited to 100–200 microns at most (i.e., two to four muscle fiber diameters)? What factors limit sprouting and reinnervation (age? sex? fascicular boundaries?) and what factors promote sprouting? We recently showed, for example, that thyrotrophin-releasing hormone deficiency limits sprouting and reinnervation of rat foot muscles denervated by local injection of botulinum toxin [23,24]. Answers to these questions will have direct relevance to the management of patients recovering from denervating diseases.

Once the motor unit has passed through this stage of reinnervation, it was formerly thought that a stage of stabilization occurred. Muscles were either fully or partially reinnervated within a year or two of the initial illness, but once that time period passed, the resultant enlarged surviving motor units remained the same. We now know that this period is much more dynamic. First of all, there is some evidence that even with full reinnervation of a muscle, there is some persistent reshaping of motor units that goes on for some time [25]. The reason for this is unclear but might be an attempt by the organism to attain a more even distribution or burden of muscle fibers among the surviving AHCs. Secondly, age-related changes over years are engrafted onto this chronic, relatively stable period. Not only is reinnervation hampered by advancing age, but AHCs are lost as age increases, especially after the sixth decade [26]. Thus, the reshaping of motor units is augmented in patients with polio when they lose an AHC carrying a larger burden of muscle fibers. Finally, there is evidence of incomplete stabilization of reinnervated motor units in old-polio patients, even after several years. Jitter and blocking remain abnormal [27] and become more abnormal with time [28], suggesting that there is an ongoing instability of reinnervation despite clinical stability. There are several possible explanations for this observation, including continuing AHC loss and incomplete recovery. It is more likely, however, that the surviving AHCs are attempting to maintain innervation to muscle fibers but are barely able to support these axon sprouts due either to their limiting distances from the motor unit or to a too heavy existing burden on that motor unit. The result is either lack of full maturation of these critical motor unit sprouts or a continuous cycle of sprout degeneration and regeneration with lack of establishment of adequate, firm contacts to these muscle fibers. This would explain the presence of unstable, complex motor unit potentials in stable patients and the presence of fresh fibrillation potentials.

LATE SYMPTOMS OF POLIO AND EMG STUDIES

In this setting, late symptoms that polio patients develop are often difficult to interpret electrophysiologically. Frequently, these symptoms are related to prosaic causes such as compression neuropathies, radiculopathies, or other common neuromuscular problems. In some cases, these processes can have a drastic effect. One of our patients had severe polio with subsequent complete paralysis of the legs and severe involvement of the arms. Although hand strength was fairly good bilaterally, he had useful proximal muscle strength in only the right arm. He then developed a right C-5 radiculopathy due to degenerative cervical spine disease and lost the use of his right shoulder, which ended his independence. Use of crutches, braces, and so forth in these patients with atrophic limbs makes compression neuropathies (carpal tunnel syndrome, ulnar neuropathies) frequent. Discovering these abnormalities in the face of widespread atrophy and marked underlying EMG changes due to the old polio can be a daunting task, and considerable skill and clinical experience is required. However, when these processes are eliminated, there remains a group of patients with late progression of neuromuscular symptoms and late atrophy of affected limbs. This is the group that is of most concern at present.

When these patients were first described, it was assumed that evidence of progressive disease would be readily detected. Indeed, it was suggested that the presence of large (fresh) fibrillation and fasciculation potentials and complex, unstable motor unit potentials was evidence of recent denervation, accounting for the symptoms [6,29]. Large fibrillation potentials generally imply that the generator (the denervated muscle fiber) is also large and probably recently denervated. Small, tiny fibrillation potentials, on the other hand, imply remote denervation with atrophy of the generator and can be seen many years after polio in atrophic, stable muscles [30]. Motor unit potentials also tend to enlarge and simplify with time. Unstable, dispersed, complex motor unit potentials with late components imply active degeneration or recent reinnervation.

Studies have been reported that tend to bear out these theoretical assumptions. Mulder et al. [6] found fasciculations and fibrillations in most of the patients they studied, with widespread neurogenic atrophy. This suggested to them a progressive disease of the anterior horn cells similar to, but less aggressive than, ALS. Hayward and Seaton found evidence of widespread neurogenic atrophy by EMG and speculated that loss of motor units due to advancing age was responsible for symptoms [11]. Dalakas et al. reported a series of twenty-seven carefully studied patients followed over a mean of 8.2 years with serial strength tests, muscle biopsies, and EMG, including SFEMG in some cases [31]. Muscle biopsy and EMG findings were consistent with chronic and new denervation but no group atrophy was found (Figure 5.10). Single-fiber EMG showed increased jitter and blocking but no neurogenic jitter. Thus, they felt that these findings indicated slow disintegration of distal nerve terminals with denervation of individual muscle fibers but not loss of whole motor units.

However, experienced electromyographers began to notice that stable patients studied for other reasons also had evidence of recent denervation with large fibrillation potentials and complex, unstable motor unit potentials. Studies compared a control group of patients with stable polio with patients who were thought to be progressing [32–34]. These two groups were found to be virtually identical and indistinguishable electrophysiologically. The patients with stable disease and patients with post-polio progressive muscle atrophy both showed comparable amounts of fresh fibrillation potentials and motor unit potential changes that were similar in nature and degree. In addition, SFEMG results were equally abnormal in progressing and stable patients [33,34]. Increased fiber density and jitter were equally prominent in both groups, consistent with the idea that motor units in stable old polio remain dynamic with ongoing change. Grouped atrophy was found on muscle biopsy, suggesting that loss of individual muscle fibers was not the sole explanation [33].

Macro-EMG [35] was also used to study old-polio patients. This technique was developed to complement concentric needle (conventional) EMG and

SFEMG and is designed to look at the entire motor unit potential. The amplitude of the macro signal correlates with the number of muscle fibers making up the motor unit (Figures 5.8 and 5.9). Concentric EMG, on the other hand, correlates only with fiber density within the effective pickup range of that electrode, a circle with a diameter of about 500 microns, while SFEMG is restricted to a pickup diameter of 300 microns. Macro-EMG showed enlargement of motor units in old polio, which correlated with the increased fiber density [36]. Jitter abnormalities also correlated with fiber density and macro-EMG amplitude, suggesting that increased jitter was due to reinnervation, not due to a neuromuscular transmission disorder.

CURRENT ROLE OF EMG

Thus, there is no apparent electrophysiologic stamp that distinguishes late progressing polio patients from patients with stable polio. The role of EMG at present is to verify the extent and degree of old anterior horn cell loss and reinnervation and thus verify the history of polio [32,33]. Patients with appropriate clinical symptoms and findings in this group are then assumed to have post-polio progressive muscular atrophy. These widespread changes are generally easy to find since patients with polio have affected muscles well beyond the areas that were originally clinically involved during the illness.

Why has electrophysiology not answered the riddle of post-polio progressive muscular atrophy? There are several possible answers. First, there may

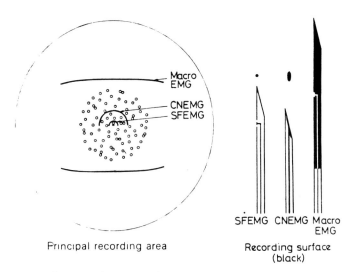

FIGURE 5.8   *Schematic depiction of SFEMG, concentric EMG, and macro-EMG electrodes and their respective pickup areas in a motor unit. (Reprinted with permission from Stalberg and Trontelj [17].)*

A   B   C

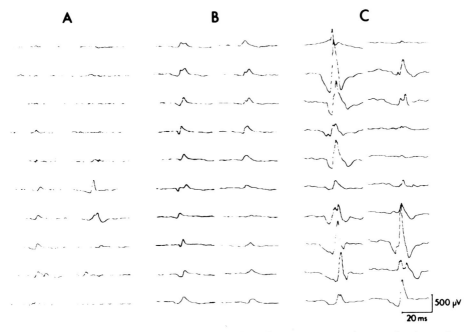

FIGURE 5.9   *Examples of macro-EMG recordings from a patient with muscular dystrophy (A), a normal patient (B), and a patient with ALS (C). (Reprinted with permission from Stalberg and Trontelj [17].)*

be no recognizable electrophysiologic change in these patients. Since our techniques are now quite sensitive, this would imply that perhaps another mechanism accounts for these symptoms. The defect, for example, might reside in muscle itself or might be due to other non-neuromuscular causes. A second possibility is that the tools we are currently using are too insensitive. Because conventional and especially SFEMG are extremely sensitive to neuromuscular change, this seems an unlikely possibility. The third and most likely reason is that there may be too much "noise" in the system because of the dynamic properties of motor units in stable old polio and the likelihood that there is some degree of ongoing denervation and reinnervation and reshaping of motor units in all old-polio patients, whether progressing or not. If true, it may not be possible to distinguish those with progressive disease from those with stable disease.

It appears that the answer to the electrophysiologic riddle of late progression of polio is not obtainable given current electrophysiologic techniques, and by standard comparisons of two groups of patients at one point in time. Carefully examined and characterized individual patients followed longitudinally for over a year and compared with matched control nonprogressing patients followed for equal lengths of time, however, are more likely to give

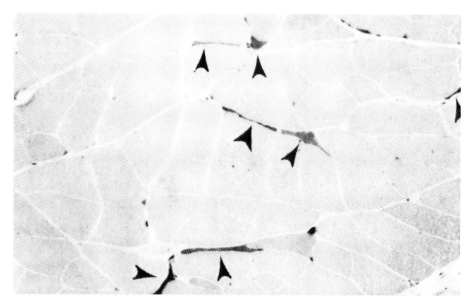

FIGURE 5.10   *Muscle biopsy sample from patient with late progressive polio muscular atrophy showing scattered, darkly stained, small and angulated, presumably acutely denervated, muscle fibers (× 125; reproduced here at 75%). (Reprinted with permission from Dalakas et al. [31].)*

an answer. These studies should include measurements of compound muscle potential amplitude, amounts of fibrillation, fiber density, macro-EMG and motor unit potential counting. All this should be correlated with muscle strength. In addition, correlating this with careful studies of muscle morphometry at the beginning and at the termination of this study would allow correlation of motor unit loss with degree of reinnervation and change of macro-EMG potential.

Preliminary reports of a few patients followed for brief periods [37–39] have shown that it may be possible to recognize abnormalities in these patients. There is a group of patients with a progressing disease who have increased fiber density and enlarged macro-EMG potentials early on just like those with stable disease. However, when these patients are followed and when they develop increasing weakness, although fiber density remains elevated, the macro-EMG potential declines. This suggests that distal sprouts are degenerating with denervation of subgroups or individual muscle fibers. Since nondegenerating branches are already maximally reinnervated, further increase in fiber density, despite the presence of some adjacent denervated muscle fibers, is not possible, so fiber density measurement does not change. However, such a drop-out of components in a motor unit causes a reduction in the amplitude of the macro-EMG potential. However, these findings could be equally well explained by the loss of larger motor units with survival of the smaller motor units. The data are insufficient so far and too few cases have been studied to be certain. Further studies of this type will need to be done to provide an answer.

REFERENCES

1. Potts CA. A case of progressive muscular atrophy occurring in a man who had had poliomyelitis nineteen years previously. Univ Penn Med Bull 1903;16:31–7.
2. Salmon LA, Riley HA. The relation between chronic anterior poliomyelitis or progressive spinal muscular atrophy and an antecedent attack of acute anterior poliomyelitis. Bull Neurol Inst NY 1935;4:35–63.
3. Steegman AT. Poliomyelitis (poliomyelopathia) chronica: report of a case, with histologic study. Arch Neurol Psychiatry 1937;38:537–49.
4. Zilkha KJ. Discussion on motor neuron disease. Proc R Soc Med 1962;55:1028–9.
5. Campbell AMG, Williams ER, Pearce J. Late motor neuron degeneration after poliomyelitis. Neurology [Minneapolis] 1969;19:1101–6.
6. Mulder DW, Rosenbaum RA, Layton DO Jr. Late progression of poliomyelitis or forme fruste amyotrophic lateral sclerosis? Mayo Clin Proc 1972;47:756–61.
7. Kayser-Gatchalian M. Late muscular atrophy after poliomyelitis. Eur Neurol 1973;10:371–80.
8. Bradley WG. Myelopathies affecting anterior horn cells. In: Dyck PJ, Thomas K, Lambert EH, eds. Peripheral neuropathy. Philadelphia: WB Saunders, 1975, pp 638–40.
9. Adams R, Victor M. Principles of neurology, 4th ed. New York: McGraw-Hill, 1989, pp 592–6.
10. Edstrom L, Kugelberg E. Histochemical composition, distribution of fibres and fatiguability of single motor units. Anterior tibial muscle of the rat. J Neurol Neurosurg Psychiatry 1968;31:424–33.
11. Hayward M, Seaton D. Late sequelae of paralytic poliomyelitis: a clinical and electromyographic study. J Neurol Neurosurg Psychiatry 1979;42:117–22.
12. Petajan JH, Currey K. Late onset muscle weakness and atrophy from undiagnosed poliomyelitis (abstract). Muscle Nerve 1987;10:665.
13. Sharrard WJW. Correlation between changes in the spinal cord and muscle paralysis in poliomyelitis. Proc R Soc Med 1953;46:346–9.
14. Department of Neurology, Mayo Clinic, Rochester, NY. Clinical examination in neurology. Philadelphia: WB Saunders, 1971, p 286.
15. Erminio F, Buchthal F, Rosenfalck P. Motor unit territory and muscle fiber concentration in paresis due to peripheral nerve injury and anterior horn cell involvement. Neurology 1959;9:657–71.
16. Buchthal F, Schmalbruch H. Motor unit of mammalian muscle. Physiol Rev 1980;60:90–142.
17. Stalberg E, Trontelj V. Single fiber electromyography. Old Woking, England: Miravelle, 1979.
18. Kugelburg E, Edstrom L, Abbruzzese M. Mapping of motor units in reinnervated rat muscle. J Neurol Neurosurg Psychiatry 1970;33:319–29.
19. Stalberg E. AAEE minimonograph No. 20: EMG. Rochester, Minn.: AAEE, 1983.
20. Stalberg E, Schwartz MS, Thiele B, et al. The normal motor unit in man. A single fibre EMG multielectrode investigation. J Neurol Sci 1976;27:291–301.

21. Schwartz MS, Stalberg E, Schiller HH, et al. The reinnervated motor unit in man. A single fibre EMG multielectrode investigation. 1976;27:303–12.
22. Slack JR, Pockett S. Terminal sprouting of motorneurons is a local response to a local stimulus. Brain Res 1981;217:368–74.
23. Van Den Bergh P, Kelly JJ Jr, Adelman L, et al. Effects of spinal cord TRH deficiency on lower motor neuron function in the rat. Muscle Nerve 1987;10:397–405.
24. Van Den Bergh P, Kelly JJ Jr, Soule N, et al. Spinal cord TRH deficiency is associated with incomplete recovery of denervated muscle in the rat (abstract). Neurology 1987;37 [Suppl 1]:161.
25. Albers JA, Donofrio PD, McGonagle TK, et al. Sequential electrodiagnostic abnormalities in acute inflammatory demyelinating polyradiculoneuropathy. Muscle Nerve 1985;8:528–39.
26. Bradley WG. Recent views on amyotrophic lateral sclerosis with emphasis on electrophysiologic studies. Muscle Nerve 1987;10:490–502.
27. Wiechers DO. New concepts of the reinnervated motor unit (abstract). Muscle Nerve 1987;10:661.
28. Wiechers DO, Hubbell SL. Late changes in the motor unit after acute poliomyelitis. Muscle Nerve 1981;4:524–8.
29. Dalakas M. New neuromuscular symptoms in patients with old poliomyelitis: a three-year follow-up study. Eur Neurol 1986;25:381–7.
30. Kraft GH. Decay of fibrillation potential amplitude following nerve injury. Muscle Nerve 1984;7:565.
31. Dalakas M, Elder G, Hallett M, et al. A long-term follow-up study of patients with post-poliomyelitis neuromuscular symptoms. N Engl J Med 1986;314:959–63.
32. Block HS, Wilbourn A. Progressive post-polio atrophy: the EMG findings (abstract). Neurology 1986;36 [Suppl]:137.
33. Cashman NR, Maselli R, Wollman RL, et al. Late denervation in patients with antecedent paralytic poliomyelitis. N Engl J Med 1987;317:7–12.
34. Ravits J, Hallett M, Baker M, et al. Clinical and EMG studies of post poliomyelitis muscular atrophy (abstract). Neurology 1987;37 [Suppl]:161.
35. Stalberg E. Macro EMG, a new recording technique. J Neurol Neurosurg Psychiatry 1980;43:475–82.
36. Maselli RA, Cashman N, Salazar E, et al. Impairment of neuromuscular transmission in patients with prior history of poliomyelitis (abstract). Muscle Nerve 1987;10:665.
37. Wiechers DO. Pathophysiology and late changes of the motor unit after poliomyelitis. In: Halstead LS, Wiechers DO, eds. Late effects of poliomyelitis. Miami: Symposia Foundation, 1985, pp 91–4.
38. Lange DJ, Smith T, Lovelace RE. Postpolio muscular atrophy: diagnostic utility of macroelectromyography. Arch Neurol 1989;46:502–6.
39. Stalberg E. Capability of motor unit sprouting in neuromuscular disorders. In: AAEE didactic program, 34th annual meeting, AAEE, October 1987.

Chapter 6

Electromyographic and Muscle Biopsy Features of the Post-Polio Syndrome

Neil R. Cashman, Ricardo A. Maselli,
Robert L. Wollmann, and Jack P. Antel

New symptoms may affect more than 25% of patients with prior paralytic poliomyelitis [1]. The symptom complex of pain, fatigue, and new weakness (with or without new muscle atrophy) is so stereotyped as to constitute a post-polio syndrome (PPS) [2,3]. The etiology of PPS is unknown, although many potential mechanisms have been proposed in the medical literature [2]. In this study, we review our experience with conventional EMG, SFEMG, macro-EMG, and muscle biopsy in PPS. Our data support Wiechers and Hubbell's hypothesis [4] that motor units grossly enlarged by axonal sprouting in recovered paralytic poliomyelitis undergo peripheral disintegration, with progressive diminution of motor unit size.

METHODS

Our patient characteristics have been previously described [5–7]. All studies compared PPS patients with a non-PPS control group matched for severity of original poliomyelitis, age, and years since polio. All patients had a past history of paralytic poliomyelitis, followed by partial or complete recovery. Patients with medical conditions associated with neuromuscular disease (e.g., diabetes, alcoholism) or patients with sensory findings were excluded from study.

Electrophysiologic studies and muscle biopsy samples were obtained from muscles that had been previously affected by poliomyelitis, but that were currently normal or near normal in strength. Muscles were matched for strength and residual atrophy between asymptomatic and symptomatic patient groups. Whenever possible, SFEMG, macro-EMG, and biopsy samples were obtained from the same muscle.

83

Conventional electrodiagnostic evaluations included nerve conduction velocities, proximal conduction studies (H-reflexes and F-responses) to exclude neuropathy or proximal root lesions, and a standardized needle examination [5].

Single-fiber EMG density and jitter were calculated from ten to twenty triggering potentials as described elsewhere [5,8]. Fiber density provides a measure of the degree of reinnervation following denervation, and may be thus increased in paralytic poliomyelitis following recovery. For comparison between different muscles, the fiber density index (FDI) was defined as follows:

$$FDI = \frac{FD \text{ (observed)} - FD \text{ (normal)}}{FD \text{ (normal)}}$$

Single-fiber EMG jitter reflects adequacy of terminal axonal conduction and neuromuscular junction transmission [8]. Increased jitter is observed in diseases associated with recent reinnervation (and thus ongoing denervation).

Macro-EMG was performed as described by Stalberg [9,10]. Macro-EMG unit amplitudes were obtained from the average of 120 sweeps from a monopolar lead triggered by a signal from a remote modified SFEMG needle. Twenty macro-EMG motor units were plotted from each studied muscle. Macro-EMG motor unit amplitudes are not normally distributed in either normal or reinnervated muscle. Thus, only qualitative comparisons in motor unit size and dispersion are feasible at present.

Muscle biopsies were evaluated with conventional histologic stains by a pathologist blinded to patient clinical status [5]. Biopsies were graded −, ±, +, or + + for evidence of remote denervation consistent with old poliomyelitis (e.g., type grouping, nuclear bags), and for evidence of ongoing denervation (e.g., isolated atrophic angular fibers, grouped atrophy). To a certain extent, myofiber diameter on biopsy can be correlated with time since denervation [11]. A normal-sized adult fiber (50–80 microns) may not show detectable atrophy until two to three weeks following denervation. Progressive atrophy of denervated fibers ensues over the following weeks to years. An end-stage atrophic fiber becomes a small (<10 microns) "nuclear bag" with little or no recognizable cytoplasm years after denervation.

We also immunohistochemically stained biopsy samples for neural cell adhesion molecule (N-CAM) in an effort to quantify recently denervated myofibers. In normal adult muscle, N-CAM expression is restricted to intramuscular nerves, end-plate regions, and a subset of mononucleated cells, including satellite cells [12,13]. Within days of experimental denervation, extrajunctional surface and cytoplasmic N-CAM is detectable in myofibers, only to be again lost following reinnervation [12]. Experimentally denervated muscle may also exhibit N-CAM+ interstitial spaces and N-CAM+ process-bearing interstitial cells [12]. N-CAM immunohistochemistry not only confirms denervation in small angulated fibers, but can also demonstrate ongoing denervation in fibers that are destined to become reinnervated before they can exhibit atrophy.

RESULTS

We studied eighteen patients with a history of paralytic poliomyelitis in order to define electrophysiologic and muscle biopsy features of PPS. Consistent with remote polio, electromyographic changes of chronic denervation were common in the 13 patients reporting new weakness, as well as the 5 control patients without new symptoms of PPS. Giant potentials and a decreased interference pattern were observed on conventional EMG, and increased fiber density was observed in four of five control patients and eight of eleven symptomatic patients (Table 6.1). Unexpectedly, conventional EMG and SFEMG evidence of ongoing denervation and neuromuscular junction instability was also detected in both groups of patients. Fibrillations and positive waves were observed in four of five asymptomatic patients and five of eleven PPS patients. SFEMG jitter exceeded normal in more than 10% of fiber pairs in all five controls and nine of eleven PPS patients, and blocking fibers were present in three of five controls and eight of eleven PPS patients (Table 6.1).

Muscle biopsy findings paralleled those observed with electrophysiologic techniques (Table 6.2). Type grouping and/or nuclear bags, consistent with remote denervation of poliomyelitis, were observed in every patient studied. Fiber splitting was seen in all but two symptomatic patients. Atrophic angulated fibers, indicative of ongoing denervation, were observed in all but two symptomatic patients. Two of five control and eight of eleven PPS biopsy samples exhibited group atrophy, a putative sign of motor neuron disease [11], although also consistent with axonal branch degeneration in an extensively sprouted motor unit. The presence of grouped atrophy was not correlated with age of the patient, militating against a role for age-related motor neuron attrition as a cause for PPS weakness [12].

Table 6.1 Electromyography Results

	Control (n = 5)	*PPS (n = 13)*
Conventional needle EMG		
Spontaneous activity	4/5	8/13
Single-Fiber EMG		
Fiber density	2.54	2.91
	(1.95–3.04)	(1.58–5.07)
Fiber density index[a]	0.68	0.83
	(0.24–1.04)	(0.02–2.23)
Mean jitter	73.7	77.4
	(39.4–120.6)	(29.0–181.7)
% Pairs abnormal jitter	65.3	44.3
	(16.7–100.0)	(0–83.0)
% Blocking	14.5	21.1
	(0–50.0)	(0–70.0)

$$^a FDI = \frac{FD \ (observed) \ - \ FD \ (normal)}{FD \ (normal)}$$

Table 6.2   Muscle Biopsy Results

Biopsy Findings	Control (n = 5)	PPS (n = 11)[a]
Type grouping	5/5	10/10
Nuclear bags	5/5	10/11
Fiber splitting	5/5	9/11
Scattered atrophy	5/5	9/11
Grouped atrophy	2/5	8/11
N-CAM⁺ fibers	3.81%	1.87%
	(0.6–12.0)	(0–5.5)

[a]PPS = post-polio syndrome.

N-CAM immunohistochemistry was abnormal in all patients, revealing staining of atrophic and splitting myofibers, and process-bearing interstitial cells similar to those observed in experimentally denervated rat muscle [13,14]. Fibers exceeding 50 microns, presumably recently denervated, were detected in all but two symptomatic patients. The percentage of these N-CAM⁺ normal fibers was not significantly different between symptomatic and asymptomatic patients (Table 6.2).

We reanalyzed our data with regard to the complaint of progressive atrophy, testing the hypothesis that patients with PPMA might constitute a separate subgroup of PPS patients. Again, no significant difference was observed in EMG or muscle biopsy findings between these patients and matched control patients with no new weakness and atrophy [6].

A significant correlation was observed between fiber density and jitter (Figure 6.1), suggesting that patients with motor units most enlarged by previous sprouting are most likely to exhibit neuromuscular junction transmission defects in later life. Notably, however, increased fiber density and jitter was observed in control patients as well as PPS patients. Significant positive correlations were observed between high-grade type grouping on muscle biopsy (+ or ++) and fiber density (Wilcoxon rank sum; $p < .02$), percent fiber pairs exhibiting abnormal jitter ($p < .01$), and percent fiber pairs blocking ($p < .01$). Correlations were also observed between high grades of fiber splitting and jitter ($p < .05$). No correlations were observed between jitter and years since poliomyelitis, as has been previously reported [4], although no patient in our series presented less than twenty-eight years after poliomyelitis.

Macro-EMG studies revealed frequent evidence of remote reinnervation (increased motor unit amplitudes) in PPS patients and controls [10]. Interestingly, patients reporting new weakness exhibited macro-EMG distributions that were clustered in the low-amplitude range, whereas control patients with similar degrees of muscle weakness and atrophy often exhibited distributions with higher motor unit amplitudes. This finding was also apparent when PPS and control muscles were matched for similar fiber density, which may provide a control for severity of poliomyelitis denervation.

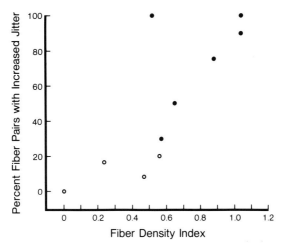

FIGURE 6.1 *Neuromuscular junction instability (increased jitter) is correlated with degree of antecedent denervation (fiber density index, p < .05, Spearman test; fiber type grouping, p < .01, Wilcoxon rank sum). Reprinted with permission from Cashman et al. [5].*

DISCUSSION

In acute poliomyelitis, death of a motor neuron denervates the myofibers it supplies. If sufficient neighboring motor neurons survive, denervated myofibers are reinnervated by axonal sprouts. Reinnervation disturbs the normal mosaic of muscle fiber types, with consequent fiber type grouping [11]. In addition, the remodeled motor units may be markedly enlarged, with motor neurons supporting as many as sevenfold more myofibers than normal [15]. Wiechers and Hubbell have provided SFEMG data suggesting that the enlarged motor units of recovered paralytic poliomyelitis may undergo peripheral axonal disintegration with time [4]. Degeneration of outlying sprouts may denervate previously reinnervated muscle fibers, which may not be reinnervated by neighboring axons extended to their limit by prior sprouting.

In our studies, increased jitter, classically regarded as reflecting ongoing reinnervation (and thus ongoing denervation), was observed in both PPS and control patients. Stalberg's classical studies with autologous muscle transplants [16] demonstrated that jitter was markedly elevated during innervation of denervated (transplanted) muscle fibers. This was thought to indicate unstable terminal axonal conduction and/or defective acetylcholine release in immature axonal sprouts. With myelination and maturation of sprouts over the following six months, jitter diminished toward normal values. However, the transplantation of small numbers of myofibers may not accurately reflect the situation pertaining to the massive denervation of acute poliomyelitis, in that elevated jitter may never return to normal [17]. Thus, in patients with sufficiently severe paralytic poliomyelitis, increased jitter cannot be regarded as a diagnostic test of ongoing denervation, but may indicate neuromuscular junction instability that dates from the original poliomyelitis. Interestingly, all of our patients had evidence of submaximal reinnervation (e.g., nuclear bags) suggesting that reinnervation was extended to its utmost in the muscles chosen for study.

However, despite the fact that increased jitter may represent a more or less permanent fixed defect in neuromuscular transmission, some true denervation is ongoing in PPS patients and controls, as indicated by the presence of atrophic angulated fibers and atrophic groups in muscle biopsies. Neural cell adhesion molecule immunoreactive myofibers, also suggesting defective innervation, are common in post-polio muscle, occurring at a rate of up to 12% of normal-sized myofibers. The percentage of atrophic angulated myofibers is much smaller than this, indicating that permanent loss of axonal innervation is uncommon. Our data suggest a hierarchy of defective innervation in post-polio muscle: (1) neuromuscular junction instability, as revealed by increased SFEMG jitter, perhaps due to suboptimal acetylcholine release in massively enlarged motor units; (2) true denervation, followed by reinnervation by neighboring axons, as suggested by widespread N-CAM immunoreactivity in non-atrophic myofibers; and, (3) true denervation of myofibers that are not reinnervated, as suggested by the presence of atrophic angulated myofibers.

If evidence of neuromuscular junction instability and denervation is as common in weakening as well as control patients, what explains the onset of symptoms in PPS? Insight into this question is provided by macro-EMG, which appears to demonstrate that patients with similar degrees of increased fiber density and jitter exhibit different motor unit amplitude distributions. The progressive diminution of motor unit size by sequential denervation of myofibers may be tolerated to a certain threshold, after which loss of myofibers contributes to the patient perception of new weakness. These studies suggest that carefully controlled macro-EMG evaluations comparing similarly affected muscles may eventually provide a useful diagnostic test for new weakness in PPS.

Acknowledgments

The authors are indebted to the patients who participated in this study, to the post-polio clinics of the University of Chicago and the Montreal Neurological Institute, and to J. Sanes and J. Covault, who provided the N-CAM antibodies. This work was supported by the Amyotrophic Lateral Sclerosis Association, the Muscular Dystrophy Association, Fonds de la Recherche en Santé du Québec, and Québec March of Dimes.

REFERENCES

1. Codd MB, Mulder DW, Kurland LT, et al. Poliomyelitis in Rochester, Minnesota, 1935–1955: epidemiology and long-term sequelae: a preliminary report. In: Hal-

stead FL, Wiechers DO, eds. Late effects of poliomyelitis. Miami: Symposia Foundation, 1985, p 121.

2. Jubelt B, Cashman NR. Neurologic manifestations of the post-polio syndrome. Crit Rev Neurobiol 1988;3:199–220.

3. Cashman NR, Siegel IM, Antel JP. Postpolio syndrome: an overview. Clin Orthot Prosth 1987;11:74–8.

4. Wiechers DO, Hubbell SL. Late changes in the motor unit after acute poliomyelitis. Muscle Nerve 1981;4:254.

5. Cashman NR, Maselli R, Wollmann RL, et al. Late ongoing denervation in patients with prior paralytic poliomyelitis. N Engl J Med 1987;317:7–12.

6. Cashman NR, Maselli R, Wollmann R, et al. New muscle atrophy as a late symptom of the postpoliomyelitis syndrome. J Clin Ecology 1987;5:11–13.

7. Cashman NR, Maselli R, Wollman RL, et al. Post-poliomyelitis syndrome: evidence of ongoing denervation in symptomatic and asymptomatic patients. In: Halstead LS, Wiechers DO, eds. Research and clinical aspects of the late effects of poliomyelitis, Vol 23. White Plains, NY: March of Dimes, 1987, pp 237–9.

8. Stalberg E, Trontelj J. Single fiber electromyography. Old Woking, England: Miravelle, 1979.

9. Stalberg E. Macro EMG. Muscle Nerve 1983;6:619–30.

10. Maselli RA, Cashman NR, Wollmann RL, et al. Neuromuscular transmission dependence on motor unit size in patients with history of poliomyelitis (submitted for publication).

11. Adams RD. Diseases of muscle: a study in pathology, 3rd ed. New York: Harper & Row, 1975.

12. Cashman NR, Maselli R, Wollmann R, et al. Grouped myofiber atrophy in patients with prior paralytic poliomyelitis (submitted for publication).

13. Covault J. Sanes JR. Neural cell adhesion molecule (N-CAM) accumulates in denervated and paralyzed skeletal muscles. Proc Natl Acad Sci USA 1985;82:4544–8.

14. Cashman NR, Covault J, Wollmann RL, Sanes JR. Neural cell adhesion molecule (N-CAM) in normal, denervated, and myopathic human muscle. Ann Neurol 1987;21:481–9.

15. Coërs C, Woolf AL. The innervation of muscle: a biopsy study. Oxford: Blackwell Scientific, 1959.

16. Hakelus L, Stalberg E. Electromyographic studies of free autogenous muscle transplants in man. Scand J Plast Reconstruct Surg 1974;8:211.

17. Wiechers DO: New concepts of the reinnervated motor unit revealed by vaccine-associated poliomyelitis. Muscle Nerve 1988;11:356–64.

Chapter 7

Alterations of Strength in Post-Polio Syndrome

R. Finkelman, T. Munsat, P. Andres, B. Thornell, and C. Brussock

Post-polio syndrome has received serious medical attention only during the past few years [1,2]. Few studies have investigated the electrophysiologic, morphologic, and clinical manifestations of this disorder. Still fewer have included longitudinal data documenting functional or strength changes over time. Strength has rarely been measured accurately, and no attempts have been made to correlate strength with electrophysiologic or morphologic data.

In this chapter, we propose to critically review past studies of strength measurement in PPS, as well as to review selected electrophysiologic and functional studies that relate to an understanding of these strength changes. An attempt will be made to identify the major determinants contributing to strength impairment and fatigue in PPS patients. The effect of exercise programs on PPS patients will also be analyzed.

DEFINITIONS AND METHODOLOGY

We define strength as the force-generating capacity of muscle [3]. Various factors influence strength, including the type of contraction (isotonic, isometric, isokinetic), the speed of contraction, length-tension relationships, the pattern of motor neuron discharge, and motivation. Numerous studies have supported the validity of strength measurements as an accurate representation of motor unit loss in neuromuscular disease [4–6].

Various methods of measuring or grading strength are currently in use. The method most frequently employed in clinical practice is that of manual muscle testing (MMT), as revised by the medical research council (MRC) [7]. This is a grading system for subjective assessment of strength and is recorded on a 0–5 scale based on resistance to gravity and the examiner's power. It is easily applied and time efficient, but has numerous drawbacks. The ranking is subjective, with large interobserver variance. The intervals between ranks are unequal with a greater degree of insensitivity in the higher ranks. For example, studies have shown that 97% of the power generated by the biceps is within ranks 4 and 5 [8]. Scores are thus generated as ordinal data that are not easily analyzed by conventional statistical methods.

Strength is usually measured isometrically and most commonly as maximum voluntary isometric contraction (MVIC). It has been shown that patients can perform MVIC with the same force voluntarily as that obtained by indirect electrical neural stimulation and with similar metabolic demands as determined by magnetic resonance spectroscopy [9]. A major advantage of MVIC is the elimination of muscle length and velocity as variables. In our view, it is preferable to measure strength isometrically in PPS patients because their efforts may be restricted by pain or by reflex inhibition of contraction caused by joint instability or contractures.

Fatigue is defined by Gow [10] as the failure to maintain a given force or power output during sustained or repeated contractions. Fatigue is often divided into central and peripheral types. Central fatigue is a result of failure of the neural drive, which may be caused by a lack of motivation or an impairment proximal to or involving recruitment of motor neurons. Central fatigue is often associated with a perception by the patient of increasing effort in performing motor tasks. It may be studied by using the interpolation of peripheral nerve–stimulated twitches or tetany during a voluntary contraction. An increased contractile force induced by the electrical stimulation implies a central component to the fatigue.

Peripheral fatigue is a result of dysfunction within the motor unit itself. This can be demonstrated by examining frequency:force relationships and relaxation characteristics produced by supramaximal stimulation of motor nerves delivered in a set pattern of frequencies. This produces a programmed stimulation myogram. Depending on the frequency producing the greatest fatigue, the abnormality may be further localized to the neuromuscular junction or the excitation-contraction coupling process. Other electrophysiologic techniques, such as repetitive stimulation and SFEMG may also be used to study the peripheral motor unit in disorders with abnormal fatigue characteristics. Although fatigue is one of the most common PPS complaints, these techniques have not yet been utilized in studying PPS.

A variety of devices are employed in strength measurement. Isokinetic force is measured by devices such as the Cybex dynamometer. This generates resistance proportional to the dynamic tension developed by the limb as it moves through its range of motion. Output is in the form of peak torque generated at various angular velocities. A major drawback of isokinetic devices is that they cannot test muscles with less than fair (3+) strength because the associated limb is too weak to move against the device's lever arm. Additionally, patients with limitations of limb range of motion due to pain, joint deformity, or instability cannot be properly tested.

Numerous devices can be used to analyze isometric contractions. Strain-gauge myometers are preferable to the handheld variety in that maximum force generated is not limited by the examiner's ability to generate resistance. Output is in the form of kilograms and hard-copy results are produced.

The Tufts Quantitative Neuromuscular Exam (TQNE) is primarily based on MVIC measurement using an electronic strain-gauge myometer [11]. Twenty-eight items, including pulmonary function, bulbar function, timed activities, arm strength, and leg strength are measured. We feel it is the most appropriate means of measuring strength in a wide variety of neuromuscular disorders, including PPS. Prior studies have demonstrated good test-retest reliability with performance variation less than 8% when tests were repeated in three to five hours [11].

Functional capacity is assessed by subjective ratings of performance and determination of disability. These scales generate ordinal data that are poorly correlated with the degree of motor unit loss. Results are seriously influenced by external factors such as posture, pain, compensatory movements, and adaptive equipment. They are less sensitive than isometric tests in assessing disease progression. If performance is assessed by timing tasks, interval data is generated and subjectivity reduced. However, significant functional loss often is a consequence of the loss of a small number of motor units and may not directly correlate with true disease progression.

ACUTE POLIOMYELITIS

Poliomyelitis is an acute febrile illness caused by a small RNA enterovirus of the picornavirus type [12]. Similar syndromes may follow infections with other enteroviruses such as Coxsackie A or B and the echoviruses. After an initial febrile illness, usually accompanied by constitutional and gastrointestinal symptoms, about 5% of patients develop neurologic symptoms. These may range from a mild aseptic meningitis to a severe diffuse paralytic process affecting bulbar and respiratory muscles. An encephalitis may be present. Following the acute paralytic phase, 60% of the survivors show maximal recovery within three months and 80% within six months. Recent cases occurring in the United States have been attributed to the use of live attenuated oral Sabin vaccine.

POST-POLIO SYNDROME

There have been a number of recent reviews describing the clinical characteristics of PPS. Dalakas [2] defines PPS as new neuromuscular symptoms occurring in polio survivors twenty to thirty-five years after their initial attack. Inclusion criteria further stipulate no prior history of back injuries, radiculopathy, entrapment neuropathy, or other systemic illness that might account for the new symptoms. Patients are divided into two subgroups: (1) those with musculoskeletal complaints such as fatigue, decreased endurance, joint pain, or increased skeletal deformities; and (2) those with new muscle atrophy and/ or weakness, termed post-polio muscular atrophy (PPMA). The new atrophy usually occurs in an asymmetric manner and may affect previously weakened muscles or previously asymptomatic muscles. Patients have developed increased bulbar and respiratory symptoms, as well as symptoms of sleep disturbance such as obstructive sleep apnea, but only if they had previously experienced bulbar or respiratory symptoms during the acute attack. Injury was not considered a precipitating event, although increased weight gain due to sedentary life-style was felt to be one. Factors associated with a greater likelihood of developing PPS symptoms, as well as a shorter latency to onset, included greater residual weakness after initial recovery, residual bulbar or respiratory weakness, and older age at onset.

Cashman et al. discussed new symptoms in PPS patients [1]. Pain was felt to be due to increased strain on soft tissue structures, whereas fatigue was considered a result of a widespread defect in neuromuscular transmission. No subgroups could be defined. Only 50% of subjects complaining of new weakness demonstrated new atrophy. Further studies by this group [13] showed new atrophy and weakness accompanied by typical EMG evidence of acute denervation such as fibrillations and positive sharp waves. Similar findings were found in asymptomatic patients who had no evidence of new disease. It was felt that this represented the sequelae of massive antecedent denervation resulting from the original acute attack.

Numerous theories have been proposed for the etiology of PPS [2,14,15]. Initially, it was suggested that PPS was due to the reactivation of the latent polio virus, much in the manner of herpes infections. Immunologic studies of CSF have not supported this concept. No elevation of polio virus antibody has been found in CSF or blood [2,16]. Others have suggested that PPS represents an ALS-like syndrome with progressive motor neuron and anterior horn cell loss [17]. However, there are no indisputable data suggesting that PPS and ALS are related. Dalakas found fiber-type grouping and inflammatory changes more frequently in PPS biopsy samples, and grouped atrophy more frequently in ALS, although these changes were not specific [18]. Clearly, PPS has a much more benign course. It has also been suggested that PPS is a result of age-associated loss of motor neurons. However, this does not usually occur until after the age of sixty and many PPS patients become symptomatic before then [19]. Currently, the most accepted theory proposes a functional and anatomic loss of new axonal sprouts in reinnervated motor unit territories, resulting from increased metabolic demand on the "overworked" motor unit [20]. This hypothesis will be discussed in more detail below.

FUNCTIONAL CHANGES IN PPS

Klingman et al. [21] studied functional abilities in fifty-seven patients with clinical histories and exams compatible with PPS and compared them with a control group of forty-nine asymptomatic post-polio patients. Of the symptomatic group, 11% demonstrated new weakness in previously unaffected muscles. They assessed various risk factors, including years since initial attack, residual disability, initial severity of weakness, age at onset, and level of recent activity. Initial and residual severity were assessed as the sum of acutely symptomatic areas, assigning one point per limb, one point for back involvement, and one point for respiratory involvement. Residual disability was rated on a 0–4 (normal to bedridden) scale. Recent activity was assessed on a three-point scale. They observed no differences between the groups in gender or years since onset. However, a correlation was found with age at onset, initial severity, residual disability, and level of recent activity. PPS patients tended to be older at onset and had greater initial involvement, similar to Dalakas' observations [18]. They had a lower mean residual disability, resulting in a greater recovery index (difference between initial severity and residual disability). This suggested that an initial good recovery from a more severe attack might correlate with a greater degree of axonal sprouting and a wider zone of reinnervation, leading to an increased risk of later deterioration. This is consistent with the "overwork" theory. No longitudinal studies of strength or associated electrophysiologic studies were done. The statistical analysis was impaired by the somewhat arbitrary assignment of severity grades resulting in ordinal data.

STRENGTH MEASUREMENTS IN PPS

Several important questions about strength in PPS remain:

1. Do statistically valid measurements of strength in PPS demonstrate a pattern of change with time, and what is its character?
2. Are there temporal characteristics of strength variations and can these be further studied?
3. Can electrophysiologic studies be correlated with variations in strength or fatigue?
4. Can functional capacity be correlated with strength or with electrophysiologic studies?
5. Do exercise programs designed for PPS affect strength, fatigue, or functional capacity?

Only a few previous studies were designed to evaluate strength alterations in PPS patients longitudinally. Dalakas et al. [22] studied twelve patients who had been clinically stable for at least fifteen years after their initial acute attack. Strength was measured with the MRC scale. Five major muscle groups were examined in each limb with a best possible score of twenty-five points per limb (i.e., 5×5). The patients were examined two to four times over a ten- to twenty-year period. A mean total loss of strength of 11.8 points over a mean follow-up period of 11.6 years was observed, averaging 1% per year. Similar measurements performed on fifteen other patients over a shorter follow-up period (mean 4.7 years) showed an average power loss of 4.1 points, again yielding a loss of strength of about 1% per year. Unfortunately, orthopedic or structural alterations that might have adversely affected performance were not critically addressed. Since the number of observations was limited and the sample group small, the statistical significance of these findings is questionable. Although EMG and nerve conduction studies were done, no attempt was made to study the electrophysiologic changes over time in the group whose strength was being followed.

Brown and Patten [23] studied seven patients who had recovery of function after a childhood paralytic illness with functional stability for at least fifteen years. They demonstrated residual atrophy, weakness, or areflexia in at least one limb and new muscle weakness with myalgias or fasciculations in a previously unaffected limb. Strength was assessed by quantified grip strength, timed ability to hold legs above a 45° angle against gravity, and ability to hold the head elevated above the supine position. Patients were followed an average of 5.6 years. The number of follow-up visits were not specified, although the graphs on two patients showed six data points over an eight- to ten-year period. Rates of progression of the different functions were highly correlated in each patient. Rates were determined as the difference between the initial and final values divided by the period of observation. The average rate of progression for all measurements was 7.0% per year. Rates did not correlate with any clinical or laboratory variable, such as age, sex, age at onset, severity, or length of disease. As in the Dalakas study, there were a limited number of observations made over an extended period of time. The reliability of this measurement system was not reported. It is unclear how measurement of grip, hip flexor, and neck flexor strength provides accurate assessment of the overall change in strength in patients who may have much more localized weakness involving single limbs or bulbar musculature. Also, progression rates based on the difference between initial and final scores is a less accurate method than that of regression analysis utilizing several data points.

A brief preliminary study by our group [24] reported serial strength measurements utilizing TQNE scores performed every three to four months over a one- to six-year period in six PPS patients who fulfilled Dalakas' diagnostic criteria. Visual inspection of the time plots of individual muscle group performance revealed no consistent pattern of change and no uniform decline in strength. However, considerable variation in muscle force over time was observed. There were seemingly random variations in strength, which appeared symmetric and often simultaneously involved anatomically separated muscle groups. It seemed that most muscle groups fluctuated in a similar manner during a given visit. It was suggested that these fluctuations represented abnormal fatiguability, possibly resulting from the adverse effect of a presently unknown metabolic or immunologic factor. This study suffers from a small sample size, which prevented statistical analysis. We are currently analyzing data obtained from a larger sample group of patients studied over a longer time course. Initial observations will be discussed below.

ELECTROPHYSIOLOGIC STUDIES IN PPS

Although many studies have investigated the electrophysiologic aspects of PPS, none have correlated electrophysiology with strength and fatigue. Wiechers and Hubbell [20] studied asymptomatic patients who had polio more than 20 years previously. They found evidence of abnormalities in neuromuscular transmission such as increased jitter and blocking, which correlated with increased fiber density. These findings were greater in patients with a longer interval since their acute attack. Neurologic blocking, a form of transmission failure seen in reinnervation where multiple fibers are reinnervated by a single terminal axon branch, was not noted [25]. These data suggest that transmission failure was originating from a point distal to the anterior horn cell or the initial axon branch point to the reinnervated fibers. It was suggested that the increased fiber density might be a consequence of increased age. These observations led to the formulation of the overwork theory. This theory suggests that motor neurons with widened areas of fiber reinnervation, resulting from previous acute denervation, have increased metabolic demand and thus may fail to maintain adequate transmission to all fibers with time. Additionally, increased physical demands as imposed by illness or excessive exercise might also stress the metabolic supply and lead to the death of new axonal sprouts, further impairing distal neuromuscular transmission. A follow-up study by Wiechers of patients who had recent acute attacks related to vaccine administration or exposure showed continued evidence of unstable neuromuscular transmission and acute denervation that appeared to worsen with time [15]. The question arose as to what electrophysiologic parameters predicted the development of PPS symptoms. Wiechers suggested that the development of symptomatology might relate to the number of unstable motor units and the degree of instability within specific muscle groups.

Cashman et al. [26] compared EMG findings in symptomatic and asymptomatic post-polio patients who were matched for age of onset, severity, residual disability, and time since attack. Morphologic changes on muscle biopsy were also analyzed. Little difference was found between the two groups with similar EMG evidence of acute and chronic denervation and disordered neuromuscular transmission. These results supported the concept that motor units most enlarged by prior sprouting were most likely to develop later instability. The study did not attempt to correlate strength with either electrophysiologic or morphologic findings and no formal strength measurements were reported for the "weakened" post-polio patients.

Feldman [27] observed absent insertional activity with normal motor unit action potentials on voluntary activity in newly symptomatic PPS muscles. Muscles that remained symptomatic and were atrophic showed neither insertional nor voluntary activity by comparison. Other electrophysiologic studies have not demonstrated these findings [15,20,26]. There was no discussion of strength measurement techniques and no longitudinal data were presented. It is possible that the absence of insertional activity was due to the placement of the EMG needle in fibrotic regions and that the lack of voluntary units in persistently symptomatic muscles reflected the results of more chronic and extensive denervation with greater loss of fibers.

A brief report by Lange and Lovelace [28] suggested that macro-EMG could differentiate PPS from other anterior horn cell processes by the presence of decreased amplitude in the former and increased amplitude in the latter. This again suggests that the origin of the lesion in PPS is distal to the anterior horn cell. However, studies by Sanders and Massey demonstrated increased macro motor unit potential amplitudes in PPS as in other anterior horn cell diseases [29]. Their studies suggest that no current EMG technique is able to distinguish between various anterior horn cell diseases, or to differentiate between symptomatic and asymptomatic post-polio patients. Although the absence of neurogenic blocking in PPS has been suggested by some as a way of differentiating PPS from ALS, it is by no means invariably present in ALS or other anterior horn cell processes.

EFFECTS OF EXERCISE

Several studies have attempted to analyze the effects of exercise programs in improving strength in PPS patients. Einarsson and Grimby studied twelve patients who had polio more than twenty-five years earlier, nine of whom developed a PPS-like reduction in function prior to the study [30]. A Cybex II dynamometer was used for both training and measurements. Isometric and isokinetic strength was measured at various angles of knee extension. A training session was carried out three times per week for six weeks. Measurements were made at the beginning of training, the end of training, and five to twelve months later. Controls consisted of untrained muscles (knee flexors) in the same patient. There was a significant ($p < .01$) increase in isometric strength measured at 60° and in isokinetic strength measured at angular velocities of 60°–300° per second between the end of training and the beginning. There was no decline of improvement when patients were retested five to twelve months later. No significant change in strength in the untrained muscle group was noted. This study suggested that progressive, nonfatiguing, strengthening exercises can have beneficial effects in weakened muscles in PPS patients. Gross and Schuch used an isokinetic training program in a single symptomatic PPS patient with increasing left knee extensor weakness [31]. There was no improvement in peak torque measured at 60° and 180° per second, either during or after a six-week training schedule. Isometric training was not part of the regimen. In contrast, Twist and Ma observed significant improvement in strength in a single patient following a program of isometric, isotonic, and proprioceptive facilitation exercises [32].

LONGITUDINAL STRENGTH MEASUREMENT

Over the past few years we have been measuring strength longitudinally in PPS. Sixteen patients who fulfilled Dalakas' diagnostic criteria for PPS have been assessed between six and twenty times during a period of two to nine years (Table 7.1). Strength measurements were made by means of a modified TQNE assessing arm and leg strength. The weakest and strongest muscle groups were selected from the arm and leg, with no distinction to the side involved. Raw data were standardized by a Z-transformation, which relates derived raw data to the mean performance of a larger representative group of patients [33]. The transformed data were plotted against time (Figure 7.1). Regression analysis was performed and the slopes determined (Table 7.2). The data have been further subdivided into groups based on age (less than or greater than fifty years) and on strong versus weak categorization. Statistical analysis was performed by t-test, comparing groups with each other and with zero (Table 7.3). Initial results appear to demonstrate a small, although statistically significant, decrease over time in the slopes, more prominently in younger patients. This suggests that age-related loss of motor units does not play a role in the deterioration of strength over time. There is no significant difference in the

Table 7.1 Patient Information

Patient	Age	Sex	Onset Age (yr.)	Latency (yr.)	TQNE No.	TQNE Time (mo.)
1	66	F	30	31	11	64
2	62	M	2	53	7	20
3	38	F	4	23	6	18
4	43	F	8	15	8	28
5	62	M	27	20	20	113
6	55	M	11	33	16	40
7	39	M	2	32	10	43
8	49	M	12	27	12	52
9	69	F	35	25	6	32
10	47	M	7	25	16	44
11	48	F	11	28	6	25
12	75	F	10	57	9	35
13	43	F	7	26	6	33
14	42	M	1	31	10	26
15	38	F	4	28	7	26
16	43	F	9	30	7	28
mean	51	9F, 7M	11	30	10	39

Patient #16 F, 43

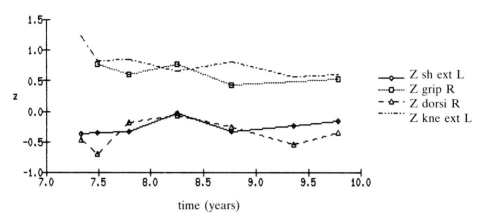

time (years)

FIGURE 7.1   *Z scores (standard deviation units) of weak (diamond, triangle) and strong (box, dashed line) muscles in upper and lower limbs over time. Strong muscles show initial positive Z scores, whereas weak muscles show initial negative Z scores. Regression analysis reveals slow loss of strength in all four functions. Z sh ext L = Z score left shoulder extensor; Z grip R = Z score right grip; Z dorsi R = Z score right ankle dorsiflexor; Z kne ext L = Z score left knee extensor.*

Table 7.2   Comparison between Weak & Strong Muscles

Patient	WUE[a]	SUE[a]	WLE[a]	SLE[a]
1	−0.09	0.09	0.00	−0.05
2	−0.07	−0.13	0.08	−0.01
3	−0.18	−0.49	−0.11	−0.29
4	−0.24	−0.32	−0.11	−0.29
5	−0.02	0.06	−0.03	0.00
6	−0.04	0.02	−0.02	−0.08
7	0.01	−0.04	0.16	−0.14
8	−0.13	0.03	0.00	−0.06
9	−0.07	0.10	−0.08	−0.04
10	−0.02	0.22	0.00	−0.05
11	−0.08	−0.01	−0.10	−0.19
12	0.02	0.14	0.00	−0.10
13	−0.22	−0.06	0.09	0.07
14	0.06	0.32	0.01	−0.18
15	−0.25	0.02	−0.14	−0.14
16	0.06	−0.11	0.02	−0.18
mean ± SD	−0.08 ± 0.10	−0.01 ± 0.19	−0.01 ± 0.08	−0.11 ± 0.10

Note: Numbers represent change in standard deviation units per year.
[a]WUE = weak upper extremity; SUE = strong upper extremity; WLE = weak lower extremity; SLE = strong lower extremity.

Table 7.3 Strength Changes in PPS Patients with Time

Comparison	T value	p value
Weak vs. strong	0.37	0.72
Weak vs. no change	− 2.74	0.01
Strong vs. no change	− 2.07	0.04

decrease in strength between strong and weak muscles, further substantiating the observations that there are equivalent histologic and electrophysiologic changes in affected and nonaffected muscles in PPS patients. Further analysis needs to be performed to determine the full significance of these findings. Visual inspection of the time plots of raw data for individual muscle functions in these patients do not demonstrate symmetric fluctuations in strength as had been noted previously when analyzing megascores (grouped data) [24].

SUGGESTIONS FOR FUTURE RESEARCH

Further studies are necessary to determine if there are abnormal metabolic or immunologic factors influencing performance in PPS patients. No serologic factors such as blocking antibodies have been identified yet, but the possibility still exists of a local factor operating in the region of the distal axon sprout or neuromuscular junction that is affecting neuromuscular transmission. It has been noted that some PPS patients show improved function with reduced fatigue when administered drugs such as edrophonium. This suggests that some patient complaints may have a basis in disordered transmission at the neuromuscular junction. Further clinical trials of agents such as these, done in conjunction with strength assessments and electrophysiologic studies, may prove important. Studies are required to see if longitudinal EMG changes showing increased abnormalities of neuromuscular transmission and ongoing denervation are accompanied by clinical findings of increased fatigue and weakness. One question that should be addressed in future studies is whether complaints of weakness and fatigue are solely organic in nature or reflect associated anxiety and depression. Correlations between self-assessment questionnaires, projective tests such as the MMPI, and strength measurements would be useful in making this determination.

REFERENCES

1. Cashman NR, Siegel I, Antel J. Post-polio syndrome: an overview. Clin Prosth Orthotics 1985;11:74.
2. Dalakas MC, Hallett M. The post-polio syndrome. In: Plum F, ed. Advances in clinical neurology. Philadelphia: FA Davis, 1989, p 51.

3. Andres P, Skerry L, Munsat T. Measurement of strength in neuromuscular disease. In: Munsat T, ed. Quantification of neurologic deficit. Boston: Butterworth, 1989, p 87.
4. Grinrod S, Tofts P, Edwards RHT. Investigations of human skeleton muscle structure and composition by x-ray computerized tomography. Eur J Clin Invest 1983;13:465.
5. McComas AL. Neuromuscular function and disorders. London: Butterworth, 1977.
6. Sobue G, Sakashi K, Takahashi A, et al. Degenerating compartment and functioning compartment of motor neurons in ALS: possible process of motor neuron loss. Neurology 1983;33:654.
7. Medical Research Council. Aids to the investigation of peripheral nerve injuries. In: War Memorandum: HMSO 1943;2:11.
8. van der Ploeg RJO, Oosterhuis HJGH, Reuvenkamp J. Measuring muscle strength. J Neurol 1984;231:200.
9. Shenton DW Jr, Heppenstall RB, Chance B, et al. Electrical stimulation of human muscle studied using 31P-nuclear magnetic resonance spectroscopy. J Orthop Res 1986;4:204.
10. Gow P, Stokes M, Edwards RHT. Investigations of neuromuscular performance in post-polio patients: a practical approach. In: Halstead LS, Wiechers DO, eds. Research and clinical aspects of the late effects of poliomyelitis, Vol 23. White Plains, NY: March of Dimes, 1987, p 293.
11. Andres P, Hedlund W, Finison L, et al. Quantitative motor assessment in amyotrophic lateral sclerosis. Neurology 1986;36:937.
12. Victor M, Adams R. Principles of neurology, 4th ed. New York: McGraw-Hill, 1989, p 592.
13. Cashman NR, Maselli R, Wollman R, et al. Late denervation in patients with antecedent paralytic poliomyelitis. N Engl J Med 1987;317:7.
14. Mulder D, Rosenbaum R, Layton D. Late progression of poliomyelitis or form fruste of amyotrophic lateral sclerosis. Mayo Clin Proc 1972;47:756.
15. Wiechers DO. New concepts of the reinnervated motor unit revealed by vaccine-associated poliomyelitis. Muscle Nerve 1988;11:350.
16. Dalakas MC, Sever JL, Madden PL, et al. Late post-poliomyelitis muscular atrophy: clinical, virological and immunologic studies. Rev Infect Dis 1984;6:s562.
17. Poskanzer DC, Cantor HM, Kaplan GS. The frequency of preceding poliomyelitis in amyotrophic lateral sclerosis. In: Norris FH, Kurland LT, eds. Motor neuron diseases: research on ALS and related disorders. New York: Grune & Stratton, 1965, p 286.
18. Dalakas MC. Amyotrophic lateral sclerosis and post-polio: differences and similarities. In: Halstead LS, Wiechers DO, eds. Research and clinical aspects of the late effects of poliomyelitis, Vol 23. White Plains, NY: March of Dimes, 1987, p 63.
19. Tomlinson BE, Irving D. The numbers of limb motor neurons in the human lumbosacral cord throughout life. J Neurol Sci 1977;34:213.
20. Wiechers DO, Hubbell S. Late changes in the motor unit after acute poliomyelitis. Muscle Nerve 1981;4:524.
21. Klingman J, Chui H, Corgiat M, et al. Functional recovery—a major risk factor for the development of postpoliomyelitis muscular atrophy. Arch Neurol 1988; 45:645.
22. Dalakas MC, Elder G, Hallett M, et al. A long-term follow-up study of patients with post-poliomyelitis neuromuscular symptoms. N Engl J Med 1986;314:959.
23. Brown S, Patten B. Post-polio syndrome and amyotrophic lateral sclerosis: a relationship more apparent than real. In: Halstead LS, Wiechers DO, eds. Research and clinical aspects of the late effects of poliomyelitis, Vol 23. White Plains, NY: March of Dimes, 1987, p 83.

24. Munsat T, Andres P, Thibodeau L. Preliminary observations on long-term muscle force changes in the post-polio syndrome. In: Halstead LS, Wiechers DO, eds. Research and clinical aspects of the late effects of poliomyelitis, Vol 23. White Plains, NY: March of Dimes, 1987, p 329.

25. Stalberg E, Thiele B. Transmission block in terminal nerve twigs: a single fiber electromyographic finding in man. J Neurol Neurosurg Psychiatry 1972;35:52.

26. Cashman NR, Masselli R, Wollman R, et al. Post-poliomyelitis syndrome: evidence of ongoing denervation in symptomatic and asymptomatic patients. In: Halstead LS, Wiechers DO, eds. Research and clinical aspects of the late effects of poliomyelitis, Vol 23. White Plains, NY: March of Dimes, 1987, p 237.

27. Feldman R. The use of EMG in the differential diagnosis of muscle weakness in post-polio syndrome. Electromyogr Clin Neurophysiol 1988;28:269.

28. Lange D, Lovelace R. Differentiating PPMA from motor neuron disease: role of macroelectromyography. Muscle Nerve 1987;10:660.

29. Sanders D, Massey J. Quantitative EMG after poliomyelitis. In: Halstead LS, Wiechers DO, eds. Research and clinical aspects of the late effects of poliomyelitis, Vol 23. White Plains, NY: March of Dimes, 1987, p 189.

30. Einarsson G, Grimby G. Strengthening exercise program in post-polio subjects. In: Halstead LS, Wiechers DO, eds. Research and clinical aspects of the late effects of poliomyelitis, Vol 23. White Plains, NY: March of Dimes, 1987, p 265.

31. Gross M, Schuch C. Exercise programs for patients with post-polio syndrome: a case report. Phys Thcr 1989;69:72.

32. Twist DJ, Ma DM. Physical therapy management of the patient with post-polio syndrome: a case report. Phys Ther 1986;66:1403.

33. Munsat T, Andres P, Thibodeau L. The use of quantitative techniques to define amyotrophic lateral sclerosis. In: Munsat T, ed. Quantification of neurologic deficit. Boston: Butterworth, 1989, p 129.

Chapter 8

Rehabilitative Principles and the Role of the Physical Therapist

Patricia L. Andres

Post-polio syndrome (PPS) is an extremely challenging problem for the physical therapist. The common clinical manifestations of PPS are weakness, pain, fatigue, and decreased functional mobility. Although the etiology of PPS is poorly understood, these symptoms can be explained, at least in part, by postural imbalances and faulty biomechanics.

Virtually all patients with paralytic polio are left with isolated muscle weakness. The human body has an extraordinary ability to efficiently compensate for weakness using muscle compensation and substitution. A secondary effect of compensatory techniques is that weak muscles tend to become overstretched and therefore weaker; and strong muscles become shortened and overworked. Over time, these muscle imbalances and faulty biomechanics lead to mechanical strain, ligamentous instability, abnormal stresses on joints, and increased energy expenditure, resulting in pain and further disability.

Since postural imbalances and faulty biomechanics are at least contributing factors to PPS, treatment should concentrate on correction of postural deficits. However, several factors make this goal difficult to achieve. First, the underlying disease mechanisms are unknown, making formulation of appropriate exercises difficult. Second, postural deficits have developed over several decades of compensation, therefore achievement of significant results in the short term is unlikely. Third, changing longstanding compensatory patterns by altering the biomechanics of one part of the body may cause adverse effects in remote parts. For example, the addition of a shoe lift will alter the forces exerted through the trunk and may actually cause new back pain.

Unfortunately, during the acute phase of polio the hallmark of successful rehabilitation was often seen as the ability to throw away orthotics and assistive devices. Thus, many patients relied on substitution and compensation techniques to achieve functional mobility rather than using their braces or canes.

This has taken its toll over the years. Long-term ambulation with gait deviations has created tremendous mechanical strain and greatly increased energy costs, which contribute to pain and fatigue.

Physical therapy treatment of the PPS patient should focus on correction of faulty postural alignment in lying, sitting, standing, and ambulating. Postural abnormalities in any of these activities, if uncorrected, can result in greatly increased energy expenditure and mechanical strain [1]. Restoration of postural alignment will decrease the abnormal forces across adjacent joints and reduce the compensatory muscle activity throughout the body [2].

Common postural abnormalities seen in sitting include forward head, protracted shoulders, insufficient lumbar curve, and/or asymmetrical ischial weight-bearing. This can usually be corrected using a properly fitting chair with lumbar support. Isolated lower extremity weakness may result in increased lateral sway, abnormal head and trunk postures, improper weight-bearing, genu recurvatum, and/or a high-steppage gait, and so forth. Use of a cane may improve weight-bearing and decrease excessive lateral sway. An ankle-foot orthosis is often used to correct foot drag, prevent genu recurvatum, and eliminate the patient's need to lean forward to watch the floor. Many patients who reported back pain and fatigue from walking are aided by use of custom-made orthotics for the shoes. Patients who have cervical pain or report discomfort through the night may benefit from using cervical pillows and a padded mattress (water, gel, or foam).

The role of exercise in treating patients with PPS is the subject of great controversy. Several investigators report that intensive, nonspecific exercise of partially denervated muscle may actually cause increased weakness [3–6]. One hypothesis to explain exercise-induced weakness in PPS is that the surviving motor neurons sprout to reinnervate a great number of muscle fibers. This produces large motor units that may stress the cell body. After decades of chronic overwork, these motor neurons may not be able to maintain the metabolic demands of all their sprouts. Thus, increased work may actually cause motor units to deteriorate even faster [7].

There are also some reports in the literature of improvement of strength in PPS following standardized exercise programs [8–10]. Einarsson and Grimby reported significant and long-lasting improvement of strength using a standardized isokinetic training program [8]. Feldman reported significant strength improvement using nonfatiguing exercises in weak muscles, though he cautioned against overworking partially denervated muscles [9,10]. More comprehensive research is needed to properly understand the benefits and risks of different exercise strategies in PPS.

It is clear that exercise philosophy in PPS has to be different than it was during the acute phase. Initially, the treatment philosophy was that if you worked hard, despite the pain, you were rewarded by overcoming your disability. Today, this philosophy simply does not work. Because of the evidence suggesting that improper, intensive exercise can actually lead to worsening of the symptoms, exercises should be nonfatiguing and specific. Exercises designed to improve posture should consist of gently stretching tight, overworked muscles combined with exercises to reactivate weak, overstretched muscles by placing the muscle in an optimal position to contract.

Management of the PPS patient must be comprehensive and include consideration of life-style modifications. Rest is every bit as important as exercise. This means that habits must change to assure regular rest periods each day. Modifications of the home and work environments should be considered to reduce mechanical strain and conserve energy.

Brief symptomatic relief of pain may be achieved using physical measures such as transcutaneous electrical nerve stimulation, ultrasound, and/or analgesics. However, the underlying mechanical strain must be reduced to achieve long-term relief. Therefore, use of modalities to alleviate pain should be used in combination with efforts to improve posture and movement.

SUMMARY

Physical therapy management of the PPS patient should focus on restoring postural alignment by (1) use of orthotics and/or assistive devices and (2) exercises that stretch tight, overworked muscles combined with nonfatiguing exercises of weak, overstretched muscles in the shortened range. Part of the challenge of working with patients with PPS is that every patient has a unique presentation depending on muscles affected, body type, and compensatory strategies, which all lead to very unique faulty biomechanics. Therefore, the key to successful treatment lies in careful evaluation of posture and movement followed by a comprehensive but cautious individually tailored treatment program.

REFERENCES

1. Perry J, Fleming C. Polio: long-term problems. Orthopedics 1985;8:877–81.
2. Smith LK, McDermott K. Pain in post-poliomyelitis—addressing causes versus treating effects. In: Halstead LS, Wiechers DO, eds. Research and clinical aspects of the late effects of poliomyelitis, Vol 23. White Plains, NY: March of Dimes, 1987.
3. Perry J, Barnes G, Gronley JK. Post-polio muscle function. In: Halstead LS, Wiechers DO, eds. Research and clinical aspects of the late effects of poliomyelitis, Vol 23. White Plains, NY: March of Dimes, 1987.
4. DeLorme TL, Schwab RS, Watkins AL. Response of the quadriceps femoris to progressive resistive exercises in poliomyelitic patients. J Bone Joint Surg 1948;30a:834–7.
5. Herbison GJ, Jaweed MM, Ditunno JF. Exercise therapies in peripheral neuropathies. Arch Phys Med Rehabil 1983;64:201–5.
6. Bennett RL, Knowlton GC. Overwork weakness in partially denervated skeletal muscle. Clin Orthop 1968;12:22–9.

7. Dalakas MC, Elder G, Hallett M, et al. A long-term follow-up study of patients with poliomyelitis neuromuscular symptoms. N Engl J Med 1986;314:959–63.
8. Einarsson G, Grimby G. Strengthening exercise program in post-polio subjects. In: Halstead LS, Wiechers DO, eds. Research and clinical aspects of the late effects of poliomyelitis, Vol 23. White Plains, NY: March of Dimes, 1987.
9. Feldman RM. The use of strengthening exercises in post-polio sequelae. Orthopedics 1985;8:889–90.
10. Feldman RM, Soskolne CL. The use of nonfatiguing strengthening exercises in post-polio syndrome. In: Halstead LS, Wiechers DO, eds. Research and clinical aspects of the late effects of poliomyelitis, Vol 23. White Plains, NY: March of Dimes, 1987.

Chapter 9

The Role of Networking and Support Groups

Gini Laurie‡

Networking is a new word for the ancient system of support services supplied by the family and community. Networking links people with common needs or goals and provides a method and structure through which they can meet these needs or goals.

Support groups are a specialized type of networking with three characteristics:

- They are voluntary, nonprofit, and charge little or no fee for the involvement of their members
- Their members are peers or equals who help each other by sharing common problems or predicaments through mutual aid and self-help
- Their members have a sense of ownership.

In most support groups, there are three basic types of activity: emotional support, information exchange, and coping strategies. The degree of activity in each of these areas will vary according to the needs of the members.

Most support groups are small, informal, financially insecure, and fluid. Members come and go as the group meets their needs. The usual pattern of their national organization is a loose network of autonomous groups. The most common is an association, supported by dues from the affiliated local branches or chapters that are authorized to use its name.

Support groups differ from professionally run groups, which are more likely to resemble group therapy rather than self-help, and they can provide benefits that professional groups cannot. Self-help groups are not meant to replace professional services, but they supplement and may even prevent the need for them [1]. Professional human service agencies and mutual help groups

---

‡Gini Laurie died in June 1989.

may have a tense and competitive relationship. Historically, professionals have often tried to co-opt mutual help organizations, and frequently regarded them as intruders.

The networking and self-help support group movements are growing rapidly, filling the gaps left by the disappearance of family and community support. In the United States, self-help groups presently involve about 15 million people in more than half a million groups.

THE EPIDEMIC YEARS

The recent development of the polio support groups for survivors with the late effects of polio is uniquely and strongly influenced by the survivors' early experiences, especially those during and following the epidemics of the 1950s.

Until the 1950s, polio was termed infantile paralysis. Children with polio learned to share with and help each other during the years they were together at children's hospitals or centers. The most famous of the centers was started by Franklin D. Roosevelt shortly after he was disabled by polio in 1921. He gathered around him children recuperating from polio because he liked company in the pool at Warm Springs, Georgia, and he wanted to share the benefits of hydrotherapy. There, and at the other children's centers, began the essence of the support group spirit.

On the other hand, some patients spent years in casts following repeated corrective surgery and felt abandoned by their families. Such mixed feelings, which were glossed over for thirty or even sixty years, are only now being faced and shared in the support groups.

In the epidemics of the 1950s, polio struck people of all ages. With improved medical management, adults with severe respiratory involvement survived. To meet their needs, the National Foundation for Infantile Paralysis (March of Dimes) created and funded 16 respiratory polio centers around the country [2].

The respiratory centers were in operation from 1951 to 1959. Contributions to the March of Dimes funded these centers and covered the expenses of staff, research, patient care, equipment and maintenance, and home care with attendants. Most of the centers were in contagious wards and directed by pediatricians who had had little experience with adults or respirators. Consequently, the centers evolved creatively to meet the unknown problems of the epidemic years.

The centers functioned as a team that included staff, patients, families, engineers, and the community. The resulting rehabilitation was remarkable. By the mid-1950s the majority of the respirator-dependent individuals went home, trained to take responsibility for their equipment, attendants, and their lives [4]. They lived full and productive lives, but not without a struggle.

In 1959, the March of Dimes closed the centers and ceased funding attendants, medical care, equipment, and research because the success of the vaccines had stopped public donations [2]. After being sheltered from all financial worries, the polio survivors faced extraordinary adjustments. Fortunately, protection and assistance were available when they needed it during early rehabilitation [3]. After that, they reacted by adapting. The less severely disabled learned to "pass" as nondisabled. Others struggled with their old braces or other equipment and worked out their own solutions. Many avoided medical care because of expense or early experiences. These were the years before Medicaid, Medicare, Supplementary Security Income (SSI), Social Security disability benefits, independent living centers, and expanded vocational rehabilitation services. The survivors had to rely on their own resources, their families, or welfare. They also turned to each other for mutual support.

FORMATION OF SUPPORT GROUPS

The survivors with respiratory involvement or severe disabilities had the greatest need for support. They had spent months or years learning to live with iron lungs or portable respirators. To fulfill the universal needs for social contact and information, the "alumni" of some of the respiratory centers fostered social meetings and published mimeographed newsletters of their at-home gatherings after the centers closed. For a few years, nonrespiratory survivors also shared newsletters from the Sister Kenny Institute and Warm Springs, and a group met as the Chicago Polio Swim Club.

Eventually, all but two groups faded away. The Los Angeles group was revived as the Polio Survivors Association, primarily for advocacy for ventilator users. The Cleveland respiratory center group was continued and expanded to include the *Rehabilitation Gazette*. The current awareness of the late effects of polio and the evolvement of the support groups and clinics is interwoven with the history of the *Gazette* into an international journal and polio network [4].

Written by alumni of the Cleveland and other respiratory polio centers, the *Gazette* became the only national advocacy organization of polio survivors, their only permanent network [5]. The publication originally was designed to share information on do-it-yourself equipment and other survivors' experiences, and to support the efforts of its readers.

The *Gazette* expanded in the 1960s and 1970s into an international journal devoted to independent living for people with all disabilities in eighty-seven countries. Yet it never ceased to maintain a living network of polio survivors. Consequently, in 1979 it was the first to notice and publish the problems its readers were having with the late effects of polio and with their physicians whose education had not included polio.

INTERNATIONAL CONFERENCES ON THE LATE EFFECTS OF POLIO

In 1980, several of these late effects were discussed with members of the medical community [6]. As a result, an international polio conference was organized that drew 125 polio survivors and physicians. Six years later, Maynard reported the following:

> I didn't know if what I was seeing in the handful of people in my clinic was typical or just odd cases. The audience [at the conference] said yes, they had the same symptoms, knew others with them. After that meeting, I was convinced [7].

As a result of the 1981 conference, another physiatrist and a polio survivor organized a regional polio conference in Oakland, California; a polio clinic opened at the University of Wisconsin, Madison; and a support group began in Buffalo, New York.

From the very beginning, clinics and support groups worked as a team, reinforcing each other. The clinics referred people to support groups and the support groups referred their members to clinics. Many clinics participated in the support group programs and some support groups arranged for a polio survivor to be available during all clinic hours.

The *Gazette's* 1983 international polio conference in St. Louis drew 400 registrants from around the world. About forty of the registrants used ventilators; most brought their own portables, seven rented iron lungs for night use. The ventilator users and respiratory specialists shared their variations on face masks and other night aids. Survivors with mobility impairments, physiatrists, and therapists shared information on the symptoms and treatments of the fatigue, pain, and muscle weakness caused by the late effects.

The conferences were also the catalyst for the support groups. They brought survivors of all degrees of disability together and revived their former togetherness and sharing of problems and information. The first two conferences reminded the registrants of their need for mutual support, and they returned home to start their own support groups [8].

The conferences brought together medical clinicians and researchers and triggered more research into the cause and treatment of the late effects. The National Institutes of Health became involved in research as did the National Easter Seal Society and the March of Dimes Birth Defects Foundation.

In 1984, the *Gazette* reorganized and expanded to become the Gazette International Networking Institute to coordinate information and networking on the late effects. The network and flow of information on the late effects of polio from laypeople to health professionals has been unique, a reversal of the usual order. Publications, such as the *Handbook on the Late Effects of Poliomyelitis for Physicians and Survivors,* support groups, and local and national publicity have gradually informed the general public and alerted health professionals.

THE INTERNATIONAL POLIO NETWORK

As a result, the *Gazette's* longtime international polio network was formalized into the International Polio Network (IPN) and the quarterly newsletter, *Polio*

Network News, and directory were initiated for members [9]. In the last two years, more than 200 support groups and fifty clinics have been started and many regional and local conferences held. The conferences have been organized by support groups, often in cooperation with local independent living centers, universities, hospitals, rehabilitation centers, Easter Seal, or March of Dimes. The conferences educate health professionals and the general public and foster an *esprit de corps* in the support groups.

In St. Louis in June 1986, IPN organized the first biennial workshop for about seventy support group leaders. Since then, IPN and its support groups have accomplished outstanding statewide organizations and systems of educating health professionals and survivors.

Meanwhile, two polio survivors and representatives of IPN eased the way for approval of Social Security Disability claims submitted by polio survivors unable to work because of the late effects of polio. Their combined efforts resulted in issuance and distribution through the Social Security Administration of a Program Circular that documents the late effects of polio [10].

Another networking accomplishment involved the Soviet Union. Responding to a request in the Summer 1985 issue of *Polio Network News,* hundreds of U.S. polio survivors wrote letters to Soviet leader Mikhail Gorbachev, President Reagan, and Dr. Armand Hammer urging an exit visa for polio survivor Tamara Tretyakova and her son, Mark, on humanitarian grounds. These letters were responsible in large part for the granting of a visa for the Tretyakovas in October 1986 [11].

The 1987 conference brought together 747 medical experts, health professionals, and polio survivors from across the United States and eighteen countries, including several from the Third World. Of particular interest were the sessions on fatigue, pain, exercise, bracing, face masks for nocturnal oral positive pressure developed by both users and prescribers, and the international exchange on independent living and attitudes toward disability. At the conference, IPN initiated National Polio Awareness Week through the concerted efforts of Congressman Richard A. Gephardt of Missouri and the other congressmen whom the support groups contacted to support his enabling legislation. A conference session for the medical directors of the polio clinics resulted in plans for further exchange through a newsletter written by the directors and published by IPN.

International Polio Network not only coordinates the more than 200 support groups in the United States, but works with a growing number across Canada and around the world through its international conferences.

SUMMARY

Support groups are a specialized type of networking composed of equals who help each other by sharing information and common experiences and who have a sense of ownership of their voluntary, nonprofit organizations. They are intended to supplement, not replace, professional human service agencies. The relationship may be competitive because, historically, some professionals have sought to co-opt mutual help organizations.

The history of the polio support groups is interwoven with the history of the IPN.* The International Polio Network was founded in 1958 as a local newsletter for polio survivors and called attention to the late effects in 1979. It now coordinates more than 200 support groups in the United States, publishes a handbook, quarterly newsletter, and directory, and organizes biennial international conferences and leaders' workshops.

The need for psychological support for polio survivors experiencing its late effects is often as critical as the need for physiological treatment. This need is partially influenced by the initial medical experience and the attitude of the public and the press during the epidemic years.

The current interest in the late effects evolved upward from the grassroots, from laypeople to professionals. There are presently more than fifty polio clinics in the United States. They work with local support groups as a team, reinforcing each other's efforts.

REFERENCES

1. Silverman P, Madera EJ, Meese A. Introduction. In: The self-help sourcebook. Nutley, NJ: Hoffman La Roche, 1986, pp 10–13.
2. Laurie G, Maynard F, Fischer DA, et al. Handbook on the late effects of poliomyelitis for physicians and survivors. St. Louis: International Polio Network, 1984, p XIV.
3. Laurie G. California attendant programs. In: Housing and home services for the disabled. Hagerstown, Md.: Harper & Row, 1977, pp 120–3.
4. Codd MB, Kurland LT. Polio's late effects. In: 1986 Medical & health annual. Chicago: Encyclopedia Britannica, 1986, p 249.
5. Laurie G. Twenty years in the *Gazette* house. Rehabilitation Gazette 1978;21:2–9.
6. Raymond J. The polio conference: a blueprint of creative cooperation for all who are disabled. Rehabilitation Gazette 1981;24:32–41.
7. Rice P. Living out the battle against polio. St. Louis Post-Dispatch, June 4, 1987, p F1.
8. Headley J. History of polio support groups. Polio Network News 1987;3:1–3.
9. Laurie G, Raymond J, eds. Proceedings of Rehabilitation Gazette's third international polio & independent living conference, May 1–12, 1985. St. Louis: International Polio Network, 1986.
10. Raymond J, ed. Social Security issues post-polio guidelines. Polio Network News 1987;3:7–8.
11. Raymond J, ed. Russian polio survivor granted exit visa thanks to polio network. Polio Network News 1986;2:1.

---

*IPN can be reached at 4502 Maryland Avenue, St. Louis, Missouri 63108.

Chapter 10

Community Resources: A Personal Perspective

Dorothy Woods Smith

Before discussing community resources for the post-polio population, it is necessary to answer this question: Who are we? In the 1986 survey of the people in our Maine post-polio support group, of the 177 people who responded, 42% had completed high school and 52% had earned baccalaureate or graduate degrees. High levels of achievement among respondents also showed outside the academic setting, with 90% employed, 81% full time. On the domestic front, we found that 74% were married, and 75% had children. In terms of physical capabilities, 63% were walking unassisted and 30% were walking with aids; 7% were wheelchair users. Of this sample, almost everyone reported new pain and/or significant fatigue, although only 12% had ever used vocational rehabilitation services [1].

As a health professional, a polio survivor who has been a consumer of some community resources, and a member of a post-polio network, I would like to share my perception of our needs for community resources, and some experiences that illustrate how existing resources both do and do not meet these needs. I would also like to offer some ideas about what may be needed to link the post-polio population with existing services, as well as what additional resources could help meet needs unique to our group.

A HISTORY OF SUPPORT

The health-care needs of polio patients were once fully met regardless of income or insurance. From the mid 1940s, the diagnosis of poliomyelitis meant that hospitalization and surgery as well as rehabilitation and adaptive equipment would be paid for by the National Foundation, popularly known as the March of Dimes. The health care assured was so comprehensive that some infants with neurological problems were knowingly misdiagnosed as having had polio so that they would receive the needed services.

When I was diagnosed at age 12 with spinal poliomyelitis, my entire body was weakened, and I was paralyzed from the waist down. I spent a month in the hospital before being transferred home to start intensive rehabilitation. During the next five months, I made several trips each week to a rehabilitation center for physical and occupational therapy, to another facility for bracing, and had a minimum of two physical therapy sessions a day at home. I also received tutoring services several times a week for a matter of months, which enabled me to graduate from junior high school with my class. The area representative of the March of Dimes visited my home, and all of the expenses not covered by my parents' Blue Cross policy were taken care of over the next four and a half years. Others who had polio who did not live near rehabilitation centers were often sent away to rehabilitation institutions where all expenses were paid. People who had polio received state-of-the-art medical care and rehabilitation based on what they needed, not what they could afford. Many have never learned to ask for help, nor have they learned what help might be available.

THE STANDARD RESOURCES AVAILABLE TODAY

In attending conferences for polio survivors where community resources have been addressed, I have found three types of resources typically discussed: vocational rehabilitation, Social Security Disability, and independent living centers. Unfortunately, many polio survivors seem not to qualify for the services offered. In the Maine network, of nearly 700 members I am aware of only two polio survivors who are receiving Social Security Disability benefits; both followed more than a year of appeals and legal interventions. One of these men enlisted the aid of a local politician who championed his cause; the other man found a lawyer who was willing to work free until his benefits were obtained.

More typical of the population is a man in his thirties who suffers extreme weakness and fatigue. When finally able to state his case before a judge, he was told that being able to walk into the court unaided meant he was able to work. Not only was the assistance denied, but his self-doubts and those of his family were intensified by the accusation of malingering.

The independent living centers typically serve the most disabled of our population. In fact, the independent living movement represents the determination and hard work of many polio survivors whose first disability was permanent, as they joined forces with others. With an estimated 25% of the post-polio population experiencing post-polio syndrome, and the rest facing potential second disabilities, it is reasonable to expect that more of us will qualify for their services as time goes on. However, at the moment only a very limited number of our population seem to meet eligibility criteria. Our Southern Maine Area Support Group recently had a guest speaker from the center for independent living in our area, who gave us information about assessments for hand controls in cars and vans; motorized devices for indoor transportation; and home evaluations for grab bars, ramps, and porch elevators. One member of our group, a full-time employee of an insurance company and father of young children, was extremely interested. Heavily dependent on crutches, he is completely fatigued by work and unable to stay awake after 8:30 at night. His shoulders and arms have become much weaker since he started using a wheelchair at work, and his 1963 automobile hand control, purchased at that time for $43, needs to be replaced. Unfortunately he is eligible for the services and equipment only by purchasing them at full price. The hand control will cost approximately $450 out of pocket, which he is not sure he can afford now that he has had to give up his second job. Nor will he be able to use the other services because his income makes him ineligible for free, or even reduced-fee, services. Although this situation is not unique to people who had polio, what it does in terms of preventive health is financially shortsighted and morally questionable. This is only one example of many who need relatively small amounts of assistance to remain productive and independent, and who do not meet existing criteria for services.

Although many of us in the post-polio population have not yet been able to use these resources, thanks to Gini Laurie's leadership there is now an international polio organization that does meet some important needs and provides a link to individuals and groups throughout the country and the world [2]. Our group in Maine, started in 1986, now numbers nearly 700. Members of post-polio support groups learn to identify needs and to pool information on what resources are available. Groups also discover what resources are not available, try to find a remedy, and decide what new resources need to be developed.

HEALTH-CARE PRIORITIES FOR THE FUTURE

Polio survivors need health care that is knowledgeable, accessible, and affordable. Professionals who provide health-care management must know about post-polio syndrome so that polio survivors are not at risk for a second disability from being directed to resume arduous exercise programs. Instead, health professionals need to prescribe supervised, gentle exercise, and to urge patients to stop the practice of ignoring fatigue and pushing past pain. Polio survivors need to be assessed for weakness and fatigue, guided in adapting their life-styles to conserve function while maintaining quality of life, and treated for spasm and pain. They need information to help them make their own decisions. Ideally, this health assessment and management would come from a team that included, but was not limited to, a physiatrist, rehabilitation nurse, physical therapist, occupational therapist, orthotist, psychologist, nutritionist, and respiratory specialist. These team members can assist by first evaluating posture and gait, work habits, and coping styles, and then including patients in a team conference where findings are identified and strategies for treatment are proposed. Also ideally this team would be under one roof, for ease of access and conservation of energy, consolidated billing, and ongoing communication.

Health professionals also need to know about post-polio syndrome when polio survivors are ill. Whether it be for pneumonia or cardiovascular disease, routine surgery, or treatment for trauma, health professionals must be aware of the risks this population may encounter with certain categories of drugs and anesthesia.

For knowledgeable health care and management to be of use to the post-polio population, it must be accessible, both physically and financially. Access to the clinic or facility should include nearby parking, barrier-free entrances, and appropriate waiting areas for people using wheelchairs, respiratory aids, or needing supportive seating. Clinics should also be close to the people that need it so that clients can visit without exhausting their resources. Although this situation is improving, the needs of many are presently unmet. In 1985, the closest evaluation clinic for me, living in Maine, was in New York City. Within two years, clinics opened in Connecticut and another was announced for New Hampshire. For some people, that still means a trip of over eight hours. The Greater Boston post-polio support group was instrumental in bringing about the Spaulding post-polio clinic. Other groups, ours among them, hope to follow in their footsteps in establishing clinics in their areas.

The clinics should also be affordable, if not free. People disabled by polio, trying to adapt their life-styles to maintain function and retain employment, have all the expenses of the rest of the population, plus the expenses of preventive care, pain control, therapy, and rehabilitative aids. In this regard, the coverage by group Blue Cross-Blue Shield health insurance is fairly typical. My post-polio evaluation, which cost $300 plus transportation, and my physical therapy, which costs $60 for a typical two-hour session, were 80% reimbursable after the annual $100 deductible was paid. At some points, the remaining 20% can be prohibitive, such as when physical therapy is required three times a week. Cost then becomes the barrier to otherwise available services. There is also the risk that new problems will be declared the result of pre-existing conditions, making people who had post-polio ineligible for services otherwise covered by health insurance policies. Although people experiencing post-polio syndrome are victims of extreme fatigue, they find, unfortunately, that working less than 40 hours a week leads to a reduction in their group insurance coverage. Many polio survivors need adaptations that could be termed preventative rehabilitation to maximize function and minimize pain. In many cases, in order to adapt the home and/or workplace to reduce unnecessary physical stressors, funding assistance in the form of grants or low-interest loans is needed. Some personal examples of relatively simple and inexpensive changes include using revolving shelves in cupboards and on desks, using book supports to read, and using lightweight plastic dishes at home. Slightly more expensive are hot packs and an electric blanket to reduce pain and spasms. Higher priced adaptations include driving a car with automatic transmission, power steering, cruise control, and power seats. All of these things are out-of-pocket expenses. There are other needs that fall into a more medical category that are not covered by health insurance since the Infantile Paralysis Foundation left the polio business. These items, all quite expensive, include a special mattress, neck traction equipment, back brace, and body cast. Some of the things that diminish pain or enhance function are just not obtainable. Not only are such things as water beds, whirlpools, computers, or modifications for a car prohibitively expensive, they are often viewed as luxuries by the population at large, including insurers and government officials. One woman in Maine was refused either reimbursement or tax deduction for a 3-wheel electric scooter she uses to get to work over snowy sidewalks in the winter. Because she already had a wheelchair, it was considered a luxury. Until the people who manage and fund community resources espouse a philosophy of health promotion and preventative health care, and these services are covered more comprehensively by health insurance, large numbers of polio survivors will continue to attempt to ignore pain, thereby risking permanent loss of muscle function.

SOCIAL SUPPORT

Polio survivors need social support from the community. Although important advances have been made in the past few years, many barriers are environmental and can be minimized if, for example, curbs are ramped, parking is reserved and available reasonably close to destinations, and elevators are well located and maintained. Some of the barriers are attitudinal. Programs to sensitize and educate children about disabilities are a step in the right direction. Toys such as puppets in wheelchairs and dolls with braces teach children that a disability should not be a source of shame or exclusion, that it is not equated with being a bad person, and that it is not contagious.

People living with the sequelae of polio need emotional support from their families, friends, and from the health professionals who work with them. Charlene Bozarth of the Michigan Post-Polio Support Group states, "People need to know that we are not lazy, we are not spoiled, and we are not kidding!" [3]. Many who are confronting existing potential second disabilities are aware, often for the first time, of the losses they have had in the past and are recognizing, also frequently for the first time, that they feel pain, anger, and fear. They need affirmation of themselves as courageous; the pain they endure is real. They must learn to listen and respect the changes observed in their bodies. They will also need encouragement to use assistive devices if these will prolong muscle function and enable them to carry out the activities that fortify self-esteem.

Self-help support groups are one means through which polio survivors address their emotional needs as they struggle with the unknown, with changes in bodies and life-styles, and with pain that affects them both physically and psychologically. The enthusiasm of one man in our post-polio support group for his new, lightweight leg brace, and the relief from pain and falling that he has been afforded since wearing it, has assisted many of us to stop viewing braces as a sign of failure and to see them as objects that enable independence. In many states, such as Maine, post-polio support groups are supported with staff and funding assistance by chapters of the Easter Seals Foundation. Some also receive help from the March of Dimes or other community resources.

Networking is another means of sharing support, providing validation as well as information. Members learn from one another, through words and through example, how to cope, which doctors are up on the post-polio research, and which facilities offer the best services at affordable fees. We work together to put on conferences to educate health professionals and ourselves, and to make the public aware of the new threat to our well-being. We join forces to lobby for services for the marginally and periodically disabled to prevent further deterioration, and to develop creative plans for meeting unmet needs.

Some polio survivors who face the uncertainties of the late effects of polio need more emotional support than the self-help groups can offer and would benefit by psychological counseling. Some of the fears they need help facing are the loss of hard-earned function and independence, the impact disclosure of the disability will have on their professional and private lives, the inability to afford available resources since the March of Dimes now serves a new cause, and not knowing whether or not they will have the strength to deal with further manifestations of polio. A husband accuses his wife of slacking off, of becoming lazy, when she is trying to learn to pace herself and not push past pain. An employer warns a laborer that his physically demanding but financially re-warding job is in jeopardy if he cannot do his share of the work. A lover expresses disgust after seeing a film dealing with the sexuality of a paraplegic. Some of these issues are too deep and too longstanding to be resolved in support groups that typically meet monthly and serve several functions including sharing information. Counselors can provide therapeutic guidance that may lead to self-renewal or personal transformation. This response, well described by Jaffe, exceeds mere physical survival, and can be eased and encouraged by resource people who have empathy for the person in pain [4].

SUMMARY

Polio survivors are trying to learn to swallow their pride and ask for help. They are working to overcome years of conditioning that they are the lucky ones, that others need the help more than they do, and that to ask is to give in. Until people who have had polio recognize their needs, consider them legitimate, and learn to ask for help, all of the community resources at hand or that could be developed will not be of use. If community program admin-istrators fail to recognize the needs of this group and realize their legitimacy, none of the programs will help. The goal, perhaps the dream, is for polio survivors to learn to ask for help, to be heard and believed, to find that the resources are accessible and·affordable, and to receive the help that will allow them to maintain productive, quality lives with their sense of worth intact.

REFERENCES

1. Post Polio Support Group of Maine, c/o Pine Tree Society for Handicapped Children and Adults, 84 Front Street, Bath, ME 04530.
2. International Polio Network, c/o G.I.N.I., 4502 Maryland Avenue, St. Louis, MO 63108.
3. Bozarth C. Psychology of disability. Presentation at G.I.N.I.'s fourth international polio and independent living conference, June 1987, St. Louis, MO.
4. Jaffe DT. Self-renewal: personal transformation following extreme trauma. J Hum Psychol 1985;5:99–124.

Index